THE LOST BOOK OF ALKALINE HERBAL HEALING

Discover the Alkaline Herbal Path for Lifelong Detox and Optimal Health, drawing inspiration from renowned herbal practices

Bonnie E. Adams

ISBN: 979-8-3302-3864-4

Author: Bonnie E. Adams

Book Title: The Lost Book of Alkaline Herbal Healing: Discover the Alkaline Herbal Path for Lifelong Detox and Optimal Health, drawing inspiration from renowned herbal practices

TABLE OF CONTENTS

CHAPTER 5   73

CHAPTER I

MEDICINAL HERBS—SUPPORTING THE ELECTRIC AFRICAN GENOME

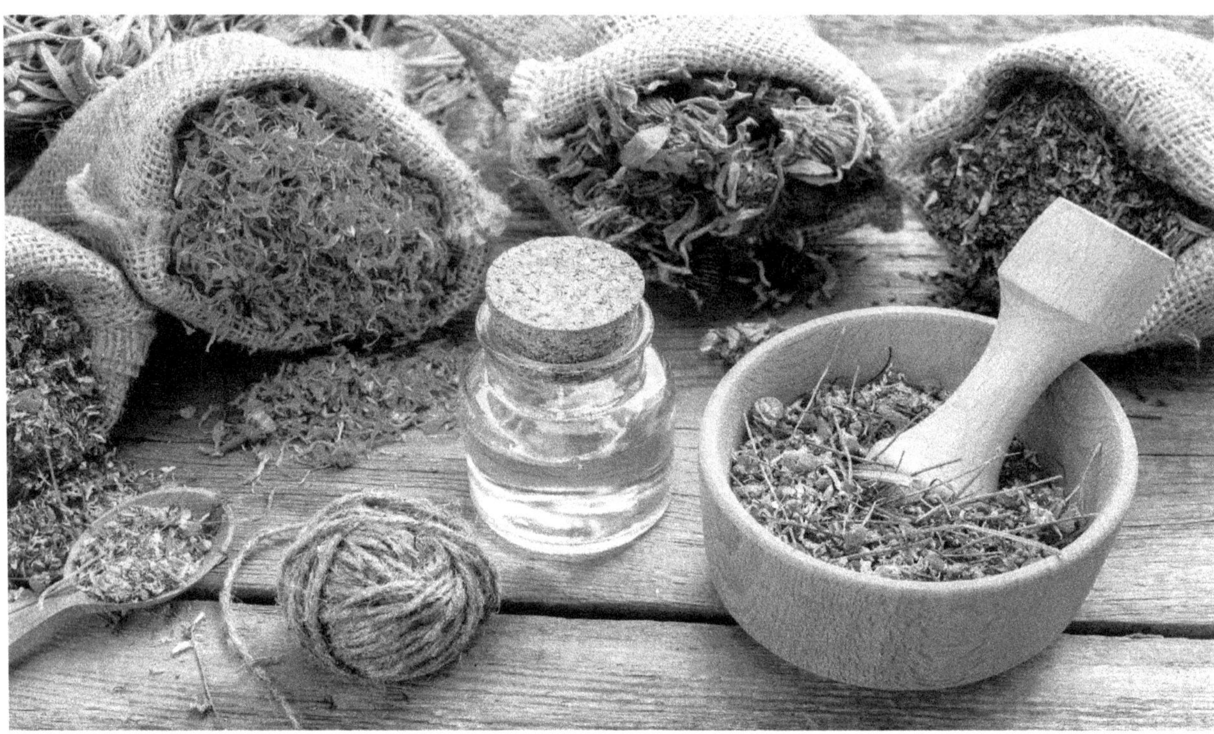

We are fortunate to inhabit a remarkable ecosystem that plays a crucial role in sustaining all forms of life. When considering life, our minds are naturally drawn to the prominent elements that surround us, such as individuals, creatures, flora, and vegetation. There is so much more to life than what meets the eye, and it is filled with countless organisms that often go unnoticed. Abundant microorganisms play a crucial role in maintaining the larger ecosystem. There exists a natural equilibrium of microorganisms that are classified as either beneficial or harmful, which can be found in our surroundings.

The larger aspects of life, such as individuals and creatures, arise from responses to the equilibrium of smaller elements, or the interplay between beneficial and harmful bacteria. The microbial balance is influenced by the intricate harmony within the earth's ecosystem and the wider universe, which also extends to our bodies. It maintains a delicate equilibrium between positive and negative forces, even at the atomic level and beyond. I have referred to this intelligent order as God/the Source/Nature in an attempt to encompass all perspectives that acknowledge this order in some form.

This intricate order that creates a delicate balance between opposing forces is responsible for generating the energy that drives the various dynamics within the ecosystem and all living beings. In order to maintain optimal health, it is important to consume a specific combination and ratio of nutrients that support the metabolic processes of organs. This is determined by the African genome, which plays a crucial role in maintaining the body's energy levels. It has been determined that the African genome serves as the foundational genome for all Homo sapiens, or modern individuals. The optimal manifestation of the African genome found in all individuals is attained through a specific mechanism, guided by a higher power or the forces of nature. Gaining a deeper comprehension of this process can be facilitated by studying the workings of an ecosystem.

ECOSYSTEM

My enlightening experience into the workings of an ecosystem and its intricate and pre-established order was a result of owning a fish tank. Maintaining a healthy environment in a fish tank may seem straightforward, but it can actually be quite challenging. There should be a well-calibrated equilibrium that has been thoughtfully established.

I quickly understood the importance of replicating the delicate equilibrium found in natural freshwater and saltwater sources to create a thriving habitat for the fish in the tank.

I assumed that keeping a fish tank would be a breeze - just add water, rocks, fish, and feed them. Unfortunately, the situation took a turn for the worse, and before long, the water became clouded with fish waste and dangerous bacteria. I discovered through experience that without a closely replicated natural environment, it becomes challenging to keep a fish tank in optimal condition.

The environment required for the fish to flourish is predetermined. I discovered that every element within the tank had a profound impact on one another. From the microorganisms to the minerals, from the food to the pH level of the water, and even the oxygen level, a delicate equilibrium was crucial.

I had to eliminate the synthetic chemicals that were added to the tap water I used to fill the fish tank. The fish's health was rapidly compromised by the presence of chemicals like chlorine. I wanted to introduce beneficial bacteria into the water and create an environment where they could thrive. This would allow them to consume the compounds in the fish's waste and generate byproducts such as oxygen, which would help maintain the water's overall health. The beneficial bacteria effectively hindered the proliferation of harmful bacteria by depriving them of their source of nourishment. The beneficial bacteria also maintained a healthy balance of nutrients, ensuring the tank's pH and oxygen levels were optimal. I believe that adding plants was crucial in maintaining the overall health of the tank and the fish. Plants have a crucial role in sustaining life in the earth's ecosystem, supporting not just the well-being of land-dwelling creatures but also the health of marine life in oceans, lakes, streams, and even in a fish tank.

PLANTS AND THE ECOSYSTEM

Plant life is crucial for maintaining the health of the fish tank and fish, as well as for the overall balance of the earth's ecosystem. Similar to how plants on land absorb minerals from the soil, plants in the tank rely on nitrates and other compounds found in fish waste to fuel their growth. Plants in both environments help to convert carbon dioxide (CO_2) produced by animals into oxygen (O_2), which is essential for animals to carry out their metabolic processes. Plants on land help purify the air, while plants in natural water sources and tanks play a crucial role in cleaning the water, ensuring the well-being of life in these environments. Plants also provide a valuable food source, enhancing the immune systems of animals through their nutrient content.

The unhealthy tank environment was caused by disregarding the established order, leading to imbalance and the spread of disease. Plants thrive in this environment, effectively combating disease, restoring nutrient balance in the water, and creating an inhospitable environment for pathogens.

I noticed that the plants in the tank were more resilient compared to the fish when faced with an imbalance. Their resilience allowed them to thrive in challenging conditions and restore the natural balance of the fish tank environment. The plants' nutrient composition and their phytonutrient makeup played a crucial role in safeguarding them from the imbalanced and unhealthy conditions in the tank. The fish would thrive by feeding on the plants and absorbing their nutrients and phytonutrients. This would enhance the fish's immune system and provide extra protection against the challenging environment.

The consumption of plant life is vital for the ongoing survival of animals on land and fish in the sea, whether directly or indirectly. Certain animals rely solely on consuming plants to obtain the necessary nutrients for their metabolic processes and to support their immune system. Other animals rely on consuming animals that feed on plants to obtain the necessary nutrients and phytonutrients for their survival. Embracing a plant-based diet is essential for promoting overall well-being.

Eating plants is beneficial for your health due to the abundance of nutrients and phytonutrients they provide. Various plants and the fruits they produce have varying levels and types of nutrients and phytonutrients.

Through careful observation of the effects of consuming plants and their fruit, ancient practices were developed to harness their healing properties and promote well-being. Typically, all natural plants provide a certain degree of healing and health maintenance. Certain plants contain a higher level of nutrients and phytonutrients, making them valuable for their medicinal properties in treating illnesses, rather than being intended for regular consumption in large quantities.

Typically, these herbs have a bitter taste and may not be the most suitable choice for culinary purposes. Additionally, consuming them in excessive amounts or over an extended period of time can result in potential side effects.

WHAT IS A MEDICINAL HERB?

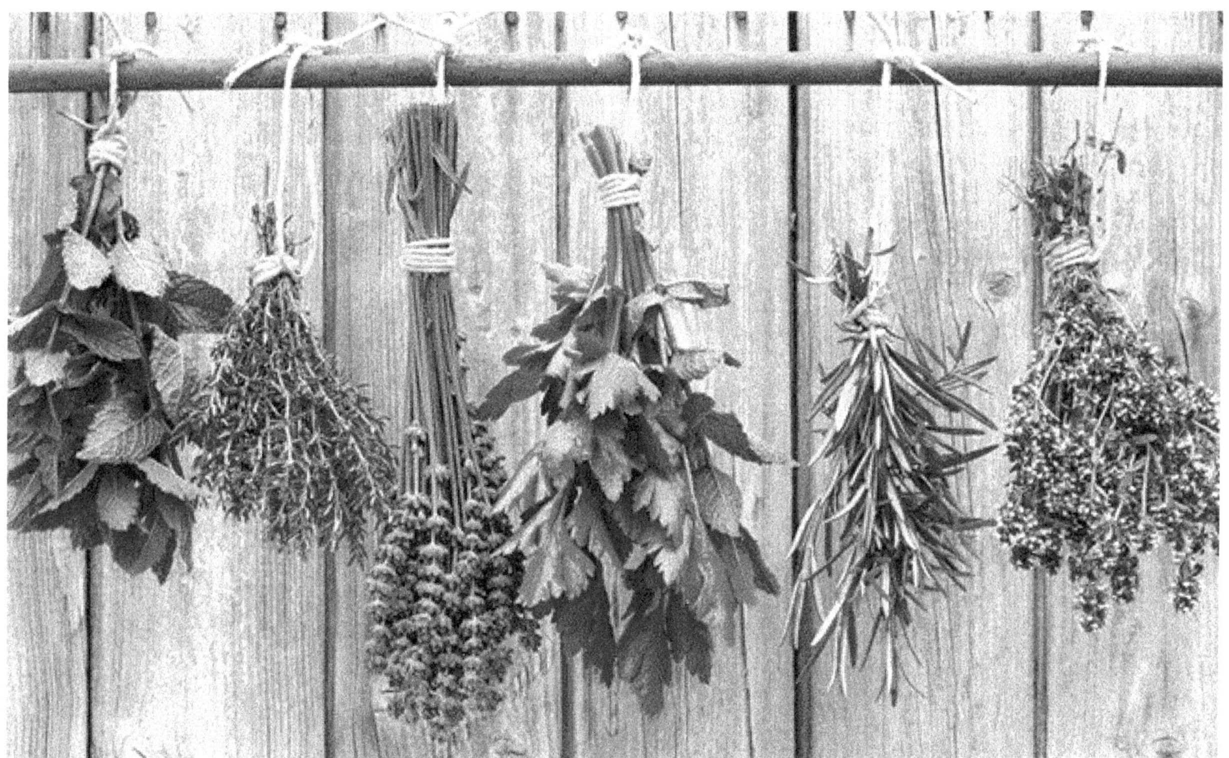

In the past, individuals had the ability to treat illnesses by utilizing natural or traditional remedies derived from plants, prior to the development of allopathic or Western pharmacological medicine. Contrary to what the Western paradigm, corporate structure, and medical institutions would have you believe. Approximately 50 percent of pharmaceutical drugs produced in the past three decades have been derived from plants, either directly or indirectly. In the past, before the world became more interconnected and certain socioeconomic systems disadvantaged the less fortunate in developing nations, indigenous communities possessed a deep understanding of their environment. They had the knowledge to utilize specific plants for medicinal purposes, offering potential remedies for various illnesses. Plant herbs have long been renowned for their healing properties, dating back to ancient times.

All plants possess a wide range of nutrients and phytonutrients that contribute to their health-enhancing properties. Medicinal herbs and food herbs, as well as food spices, have a distinct flavor profile that sets them apart from regular plant foods. This is because they contain a higher concentration of nutrients and phytonutrients, which contribute to their either bitter, aromatic, or pungent taste. Medicinal herbs such as cardo santo or hombre grande are mainly obtained from flowers, roots, and barks. They tend to have a stronger and more potent effect in treating diseases compared to culinary herbs. Food herbs such as rosemary and thyme are mainly obtained from plant leaves, and incorporating small quantities of these spices can impart intensely aromatic or pungent flavors to dishes. Due to their rich concentration of nutrients and phytonutrients, these herbs are occasionally utilized in higher dosages and are recognized for their medicinal properties in traditional medicine.

MEDICINAL HERBS AND THE BODY'S NATURAL HEALING PROCESS

The human body is an incredible and intricate machine that has the ability to naturally correct itself. It was created with the ability to combat and eliminate diseases, restore damaged cells, and, if needed, eliminate severely damaged cells. Throughout a person's lifetime, the body diligently replaces old cells with new ones through the process of cell replication. This is how the body ensures the overall well-being of its blood and organs. Many cells in the body undergo a natural process called apoptosis, where they replace themselves and eventually die off.

Red blood cells are constantly replenished, bones undergo a renewal process every decade, the lining of the stomach and intestines is refreshed every few days, and the skin undergoes a regeneration cycle every few weeks. Scientists are now reevaluating the idea that brain cells were once thought to be unable to regenerate. The body carries out these processes using specialized substances and molecules. Phytonutrients help support the functions of these molecules and contribute to the overall well-being of the organs responsible for their production. This design is incredibly intricate and clearly the result of a highly skilled and thoughtful process.

Consuming plants and their phytonutrients can help strengthen the immune system by providing the body with organic compounds. These powerful compounds have the ability to eliminate cancer cells, support DNA repair, cleanse the body of toxins, improve cell communication, eliminate harmful pathogens, and act as antioxidants to shield cells from damage caused by free radicals and aging. There are different classes of phytonutrients, such as carotenoids, flavonoids, phytates, ligans, isothiocyanates or indoles, phenols, saponins, sulfides, and terpenes, which have various effects on the body.

During the replication process, the body takes every possible measure to ensure the health of the cells. It will utilize its own internal processes and also rely on nutrients and phytonutrients obtained from plants to ensure the replication of cells without any harm from pathogens or toxins.

Certain phytonutrients have the ability to interact with specific cells, pathogens, and toxins, effectively cleansing the cells and neutralizing the harmful substances.

The flavonoids found in the elderberry herb have the unique ability to bind with the HINI flu virus and prevent it from entering cells. This sets elderberry apart from other plants, whose phytonutrients lack this capability. Certain plants contain phytonutrients that can be recognized by cell receptors and have the ability to enter cells, effectively cleansing them of pathogens and toxins. However, there are also some phytonutrients that are only capable of neutralizing pathogens and toxins in the bloodstream. Herbs such as cardo santo and cascara sagrada are utilized for cellular cleansing at the intracellular level.

MEDICINAL HERBS FOR THE ELECTRIC GENOME OF HOMO SAPIENS

The African body is a prime example of human development. The origin of human life can be traced back to Africa, from where it gradually dispersed to various regions across the globe. Regardless of your beliefs in evolution, religion, or a combination of both, a thorough and impartial analysis will point to Africa as the origin of the human journey. Africa has played a crucial role in shaping the modern human lineage across the globe. After years of research and analysis, evolutionary science has made a significant breakthrough in understanding the origins of modern human life. It is now widely accepted that human life originated in Africa and gradually spread across the globe, despite the challenges posed by racism, prejudice, and political and economic agendas.

THE ELECTRIC AFRICAN GENOME AND BODY

The environment in Africa provides optimal conditions for the African genome, which serves as the basis for all human life. The environment encompasses various factors such as the impact of sunlight on life, the composition of the air and its equilibrium, and the presence of minerals and compounds in the soil. Microorganisms, plant life, animal life, and human life evolved in unique ways as a result of their close relationship with the African ecosystem. Remove an element, and life takes a different course.

Introduce an element, and life takes a different path. The interaction between Africans and the African ecosystem resulted in the development of a body that possessed strong electrical and alkaline properties.

This enhanced the Africans' physical and mental well-being and connected them with the healing environment of the African ecosystem.

The African body maintains a state of homeostasis that is determined by its genetic makeup. Homeostasis is the ideal state in which all of the body's organs function at their best. It is possible that this genetic structure evolved in response to the African ecosystem, or it may have been influenced by a higher power I like to call God/the Source/Nature. I came up with the term God/the Source/Nature in an effort to encompass all perspectives that acknowledge this inherent order in life, in various ways.

The environmental factors in Africa and the overall lifestyle contributed to maintaining a balanced state of homeostasis in the body. The plant-centered diets of the early Africans, which prioritized the consumption of alkaline plants, naturally promoted the electrical balance and healthy expression of the African genome. Examining this topic from a scientific standpoint, it is believed that African humans have evolved from great apes, which primarily consumed plants. The great apes have a natural inclination towards consuming predominantly plant-based foods due to their genetic makeup. It is believed that humans have a natural inclination towards consuming a plant-based diet in order to promote the optimal expression of their genetic makeup. Africa's environment, characterized by its consistently warm climate, facilitated the year-round growth of plant food. The consumption of meat was introduced by Neanderthals as they adapted to their less hospitable environment. This came with a cost of the negative impact on the African genome, including the manifestation of diseases and genetic mutations.

The plant life that thrived in Africa flourished in the same environmental conditions as the African ecosystem. It was created with a broader range of nutrients and a complete structure that had a chemical affinity with the African genome. These plants were consumed without causing any negative effects on the body's well-being or disrupting its balance. The natural plant foods and herbs greatly contributed to the optimal expression of the African genome, promoting overall health and well-being. These natural plant foods were of exceptional quality, with a perfect balance of carbohydrates, fats, proteins, vitamins, and minerals. They contributed to a highly charged state in the body, promoting optimal physical, mental, and emotional well-being.

Flowers with medicinal properties that originated outside Africa also played a role in supporting the African genome. They might have been more resilient in certain aspects due to the need to develop their phytonutrients to survive in harsher environmental conditions. The chilly climate and limited sunlight in the area hindered the continuous cultivation of medicinal herbs.

Natural plants are plants that have not been altered by human intervention. A significant number of the plants consumed nowadays are a product of human intervention, where two or more plants have been crossbred. This has a detrimental impact on the natural nutrient balance in plants, leading to increased acidity and disrupting the body's homeostasis and electrical activity.

The state of homeostasis determined by the African genome was highly electric, with the consumption of natural plant foods providing the necessary nutrients to support optimal energy transmission throughout the body. Optimal charging of the body's "battery" can be achieved by consuming a diet rich in natural plants. Similar to a battery, the body's strength or electrical charge diminishes with use. Fortunately, the body operates like a rechargeable battery, replenishing itself with the necessary nutrients when consuming natural plants.

Our bodies rely on electrical signals transmitted through the nervous system to control various functions, including thinking, muscle contraction, and fluid movement. The nervous system functions as a bidirectional system, facilitating the transmission of electrical signals between the brain and all organs in the body.

These signals effortlessly travel from cell to cell until the messages reach their destination, and these messages are delivered almost instantaneously under normal circumstances. The body can generate this electricity through the interaction of electrolytes.

Electrolytes are compounds that undergo ionization and acquire either a positive or negative charge when they interact with water in the body. This leads to the formation of ions with positive charges (cations) such as calcium, magnesium, potassium, or sodium, and ions with negative charges (anions) like chloride or phosphorous. The generation of electricity is a direct result of the movement and interaction of positive and negative electrolytes across cell membranes.

Electrolytes are essential for maintaining a healthy heart, supporting metabolic processes within cells, ensuring proper organ function, and enabling muscle activity.

Electrolytes play a crucial role in maintaining the body's health and vitality, with the kidneys working tirelessly to ensure the optimal balance of these essential substances in the blood. Excess fat can significantly hinder the optimal flow of electricity in the body. Electricity travels more efficiently through water than through fat, which can hinder its ability to rapidly transmit impulses to the necessary areas in the body. Diets focused on whole plant foods provide fat in the diet at approximately 10 percent of the calories consumed. This percentage naturally ensures an optimal fat ratio to support metabolic processes and facilitate the smooth transmission of electrical messages throughout the body.

Not only do natural plant foods provide electrolytes and nutrients that are more beneficial for the healthy expression of the African genome, but their composition also tends to be more alkaline on the pH scale. This was ideal for maintaining a slightly alkaline blood pH level of around 7.4, as the body actively regulates its acidity. Consuming an excess of acidic foods, such as meat, dairy, and processed foods, can lead to the body extracting alkaline substances from other parts of the body, like bones, in order to maintain a slightly alkaline bloodstream. An alkaline environment in the blood promotes optimal oxygenation of cells and facilitates metabolic processes. This also promotes a strong immune system that actively targets and eliminates harmful pathogens and toxins.

Africa's abundant plant life provided the African people with the perfect balance of nutrients to fuel their bodies and promote optimal physical and mental well-being. This natural source of sustenance contributed to their high energy levels and overall vitality.

NEANDERTHAL GENOME

The most recent evolutionary model recognizes Africans in Africa as genuine Homo sapiens. It is widely believed that Neanderthals and African Homo sapiens shared a common ancestor, although their genetic makeup differed slightly. Genetic scientists have successfully isolated unique genetic information found exclusively in Neanderthals and Denisovans, which is absent in Africans due to their lack of intermixing.

According to a widely accepted scientific model, it is believed that African Homo sapiens, Neanderthals, and Denisovans all originated from a common ancestor and evolved separately. There is another theory suggesting that Homo heidelbergensis, an ancient human species, once resided in Africa. It is believed that a portion of this group departed Africa around two to three hundred thousand years ago, and later divided into separate groups. The Africans who stayed in Africa evolved into Homo sapiens. The group that migrated from Africa eventually evolved into Neanderthals, who made their homes in the caves of the Neandertal, a picturesque river valley in Germany. The Neanderthals, who later separated from their group, migrated towards the east into Asia and underwent further genetic changes, resulting in the emergence of the lesser-known Denisovan hominid. It is probable that Neanderthals and Denisovans emerged from a mutation of the African genome, rather than all three arising from a common ancestor.

The DNA of Neanderthals and Denisovans includes genetic information from Africa and other sources. If Neanderthals and Denisovans had a common ancestor with Homo sapiens, it would be expected that the Homo sapiens genome would possess distinct information compared to that of Neanderthals and Denisovans. It seems that the African Homo sapiens genome is the key factor, while other information in the genome led to the emergence of the Neanderthals and Denisovans.

Scientific evidence suggests that the genomes of Neanderthals and Denisovans were discovered outside of Africa, indicating that these genomes originated beyond the borders of Africa. It is probable that the environmental conditions outside of Africa have had an impact on the way the African genome has evolved over a long period of time.

The African genome has been shaped by its interactions with the European and East Asian environments over an extensive period of time. This is probably why the Neanderthal and Denisovan genomes were developed. The harsh conditions greatly influenced the African genome's expression and likely brought about modifications.

For example, people in Africa typically experienced a warm and sunny climate. Africans have a higher concentration of melanin in their skin, which serves as a natural defense against the harmful effects of UV radiation from the sun. This could have arisen through natural processes over time or been intentionally created. Given the higher exposure to sunlight, Africans developed a greater amount of melanin to provide enhanced protection. The melanin helps regulate the absorption of UV rays, leading to a gradual production of vitamin D in the blood over time.

Due to the harsh conditions of their environment, Neanderthals evolved proteins that strengthened their skin, enabling them to withstand the cold climate more effectively. They also lost their melanin and the natural protection against UV rays. They were able to produce vitamin D at a faster rate when exposed to the sun. Their offspring inherited these variations through their inherited genes, which supports the idea that the environment can influence gene expression. It is crucial to gain a comprehensive understanding of the potential manifestations of the variations between the African Homo sapiens genome and the Neanderthal genome.

The genetic scientists and authors of the Neanderthal ancestry study discovered genetic variants linked to various health conditions such as lupus, biliary cirrhosis, Crohn's disease, optic-disk size, and type 2 diabetes. They also identified certain behaviors, like the ability to quit smoking that may be influenced by these genetic factors. Through countless years of interaction between the African body and the European environment, a unique genetic makeup emerged, making individuals more prone to certain illnesses.

The Neanderthals resided in caves in the Neander Valley and relied heavily on a meat-based diet. This was due to the limitations of their environment, which did not provide abundant and diverse vegetation throughout the year. The plant life that thrived in Europe's challenging conditions faced colder temperatures and nutrient-deficient soil, unlike the more favorable environments found in Africa, the Caribbean, and Central and South America. The lifestyle and environment of the Neanderthals did not adequately support the optimal expression of the African genome, leading to a higher susceptibility to disease.

Africans embarked on another migration out of Africa approximately thirty thousand years ago. As Africans migrated, they established their own communities in various regions beyond Africa, where they encountered Neanderthals and Denisovans. Neanderthals and Denisovans are no longer present in our world today. It has been suggested that the phenomenon of natural selection resulted in reproductive challenges for these ancient human species, ultimately leading to their demise. A fascinating revelation emerges from DNA analysis, revealing the intricate intermingling of African and Neanderthal/Denisovan ancestry. This intricate genetic exchange gave rise to hybrid populations in Europe and Eastern Asia, bridging the gap between different human lineages.

The African genome is a common aspect shared by the African, African/Neanderthal, and African/Denisovan peoples. As Africans intermixed with the African/Neanderthals and African/Denisovans, the reintroduction of the complete African genome had a positive impact on stabilizing the mutations and promoting a healthier expression of the African genome in these populations. In order to develop a highly electric and healthy body, it is important to fully express the African genome. This can be achieved by following a diet that focuses on consuming natural plant foods and herbs that have chemical affinities with the African genome.

Meat-based diets and environmental factors are believed to have played a significant role in the evolution of the African genome over a long period of time. This evolution eventually led to the emergence of the Neanderthal and Denisovan genomes, which carry genetic markers associated with certain diseases.

HEALTHY EXPRESSION OF THE COMMON AFRICAN GENOME

To fully support the optimal expression of the African genome, which is crucial for human life, it is important to consider adopting a plant-centered diet. This dietary choice promotes overall health and avoids the negative effects associated with conditions that influenced the Neanderthal. Plant-centered diets primarily consist of plant foods, although they may include some non-plant foods as well. Meat was occasionally consumed as a small part of a plant-centered diet. Plant-centered diets were widely adopted in Africa and other regions with similar environments, such as Central and South America, the Caribbean, and India. These diets were found to have a positive impact on the expression of the African genome, promoting overall health. Deviating from this diet, like the Neanderthals did, resulted in the manifestation of health issues and diseases in the African genome.

Opting for a plant-based diet, which consists solely of plant foods, is proven to be more beneficial for maximizing the health potential of the African genome. Emphasizing the significance of a plant-based diet and incorporating plant herbs is crucial for combating disease. By reducing the intake of toxins and unhealthy substances found in meat, these dietary choices promote the optimal functioning of the African genome. Consuming plants has been ingrained in the African genome, promoting a healthy expression of the genome and leading to stability in physical, mental, and emotional well-being. The challenging conditions of the European environment and a diet focused on meat consumption resulted in the manifestation of the Neanderthal genome and the related diseases.

Consuming plants is crucial for maintaining a healthy genome, as natural plants have a strong chemical connection with it, making them the most effective support. The genome enables the body to efficiently process natural plants due to their chemical composition, which promotes the healthy expression of the genome and prevents the onset of diseases. The favorable conditions found in Africa and similar environments, including nutrient-rich soil, nurturing weather, and abundant sunshine, fostered the development of a robust and thriving African genome. In this particular setting, the conditions fostered the growth of plant life that possessed fully-formed structures and genetic profiles that aligned with the African genome, promoting well-being rather than illness.

Plants contribute to the well-being of the body in two distinct ways. Firstly, they offered a diverse range of minerals, vitamins, carbohydrates, fats, and protein in proportions that naturally aligned with the body's nutrient ratios. The body efficiently utilized the nutrients to replenish the ones expended during metabolic processes that sustain organ function. Additionally, the body can harness the unique and diverse chemical compounds found in plants, which plants naturally produce to defend against diseases. Africa and other similar environments have a rich abundance of plants that naturally thrive and provide ample supply.

There are certain plants that thrive in challenging environments beyond Africa, which could potentially provide a diverse array of nutrients. They frequently include phytonutrients that provide protection against a range of diseases. Certain plants possess remarkable resilience and can thrive in extremely challenging environments due to their phytonutrients. These plants are frequently sought after for their valuable medicinal qualities. These plants are commonly known as weeds due to their remarkable ability to thrive in unwanted conditions. The presence of natural plants in various environments contributes to the overall well-being of the body.

The combination of different plant species disrupts their natural chemical balance, leading to an increased risk of disease instead of promoting overall health and proper functioning of the body's organs and metabolic processes. When multiple hybridizations are performed, there is a higher risk of creating compounds that do not interact well with the body, despite the hybridized plants still retaining some nutritional value. We must prioritize the consumption of natural plants, both as food and as herbs, to fully support the healthy expression of the African genome, which is essential for the well-being of all individuals.

It is highly beneficial for individuals, including Africans and their descendants, to prioritize the consumption of plant-centered diets and even plant-based diets that consist of natural nonhybrid plants. This dietary choice can greatly contribute to enhancing physical, mental, and emotional well-being. Africans have adopted a variety of culinary influences due to historical events such as slavery, colonialism, and globalization. It is clear that the Western diet contributes to the onset of chronic illnesses, which are also linked to the Neanderthal genome. European history has seen a higher prevalence of chronic diseases when compared to Africa and similar countries prior to the era of colonialism and slavery. The widespread adoption of a diet centered around meat, along with the inclusion of genetically modified plants and processed foods, is having a detrimental impact on our health. To achieve optimal well-being, it is important to eliminate the consumption of these foods and instead focus on nourishing our bodies with natural plants and their nutrients, which are gifts from the divine/the universe/nature. These plants possess unique properties that can aid in the restoration of health and promote the optimal functioning of the African genome. It has been acknowledged by the scientific community that certain individuals may have a genetic predisposition that increases their susceptibility to a particular disease. However, scientific evidence also suggests that environmental factors, such as diet, have a more significant impact on how genes are expressed and the likelihood of developing chronic illnesses.

Animals and plants in Africa, Europe, and East Asia developed differently due to the variations in their environments. Africa's rich natural resources and abundant sunshine fostered the growth of a vibrant and energetically charged life. The vibrant interaction between the sun and the abundant natural elements in the environment fostered the development of life that thrived with those minerals, enhancing both mental and physical vitality.

CHAPTER 2

ALKALINE PLANT FOOD

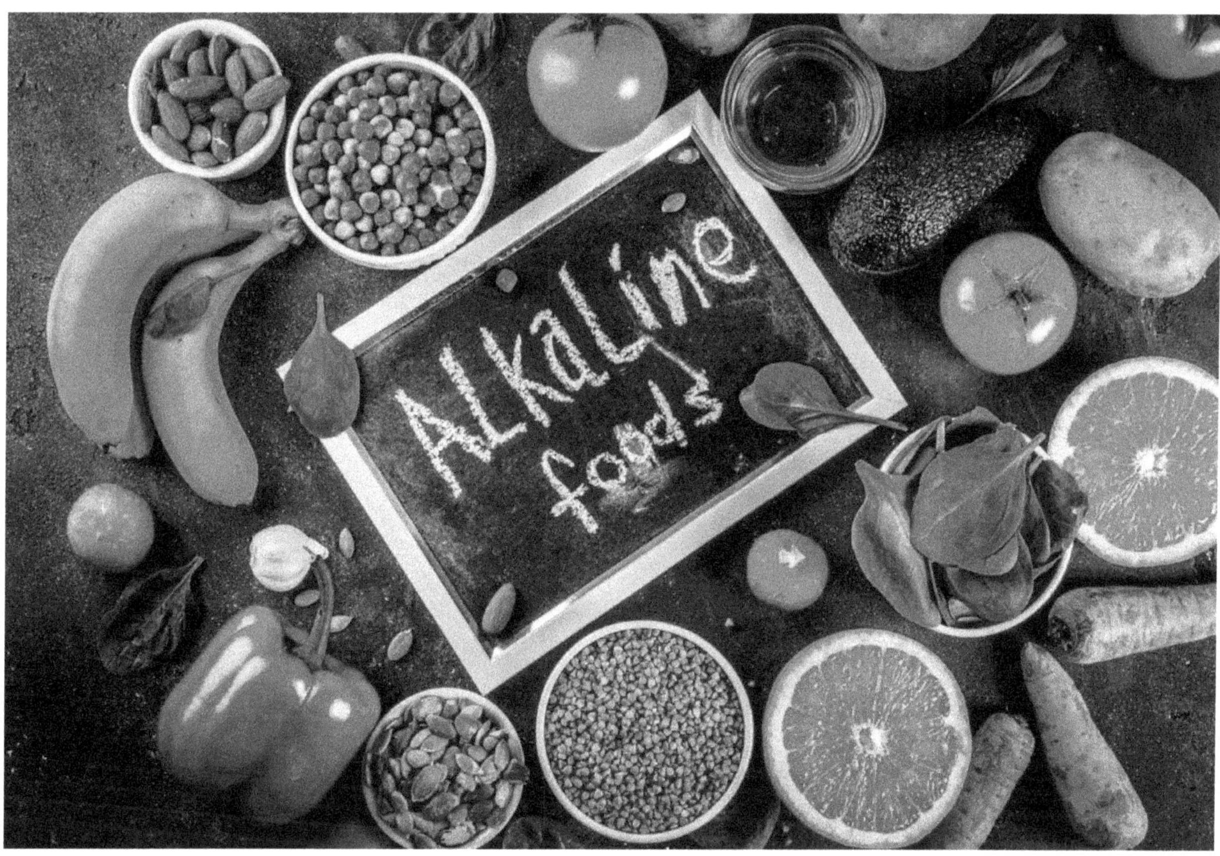

It is important to shift the focus of the Western diet, which is becoming increasingly globalized, away from meat, dairy, processed foods, and hybridized and genetically modified plant foods. Instead, we should prioritize a diet that revolves around the consumption of alkaline plant foods. We should consider exploring plant foods that are native to Africa or other regions with similar environmental conditions, such as Central and South America, the Caribbean, and India. These foods thrive in the conditions that have nurtured the African genome and the plants that share chemical affinities with it, forming the basis of the human genome in all individuals.

Begin the healing process by eliminating foods that introduce harmful substances and pathogens into the body, resulting in acidification, mucus accumulation, chronic inflammation, and the onset of chronic illnesses. A report from the World Health Organization (WHO) has classified the consumption of processed meat as "carcinogenic to humans" and the consumption of red meat as "probably carcinogenic to humans." There is a wealth of scientific research that strongly suggests a link between the consumption of animal protein and fat, and an increased risk of developing chronic diseases such as cancer, heart disease, and diabetes.

In order to promote the healing process and maintain balance in the body, it is important to focus on a diet that consists primarily of unprocessed, plant-based foods. This forms the basis for optimal health and the process of healing. To enhance the healing process or address intricate health conditions, it is advisable to incorporate the use of natural alkaline non-hybrid plant herbs.

An esteemed expert in herbal medicine has been instrumental in reintroducing the idea that alkaline, non-hybrid plant foods possess chemical affinities with the body and can contribute to healing. The healing methodology I'm referring to is based on the idea that specific types of food can raise the acidity level in the body and result in excessive mucus production, which is thought to be the root cause of illness. Basically, the body is constantly being targeted by acidic and toxin-filled foods, leading to a long-lasting inflammatory response and the emergence of chronic inflammation.

Acute inflammation is a vital process that the body uses to combat infection and heal physical damage. When acute inflammation persists, it can harm healthy cells in different parts of the body, potentially causing the onset of various diseases. This affects the protective mucous membrane that lines the organs and leads to an increase in mucus production, which in turn affects the overall health of the organs. Let's begin by eliminating certain foods from our diet, such as meat, dairy, processed foods, and hybrid plant foods that are not naturally alkaline. Here's a helpful list of foods that align with the alkaline foods recommended by this herbalist.

ALKALINE PLANT FOODS AND HERBS SUPPORT THE ALKALINE BODY

When the body becomes too acidic, it becomes susceptible to various diseases. When the body becomes too acidic, it can negatively impact the mucous membrane that plays a crucial role in protecting our organs. This can potentially contribute to the development of chronic diseases. While the body's various areas have different pH levels, it is important to consume alkaline foods to support the body's natural pH balance of 7.4 in the blood.

The concept of pH refers to the capacity of molecules to attract hydrogen ions, which is crucial for understanding their behavior. The availability of hydrogen decreases as the pH level increases. The availability of hydrogen increases as the pH level decreases. The pH scale spans from 0 to 14. The scale ranges from 0 to 14, with 0 indicating the highest acidic level, 7 being neutral, and 14 representing the highest alkaline level.

The stomach has a pH range of 1.35 to 3.5, but the "mucous neck cells" located just below the surface of the stomach lining maintain a neutral pH.

The skin's outer layer maintains a pH of around 4.0 to shield itself from bacteria in the environment, while the inner layer has a pH of approximately 6.9.

The vagina maintains a pH of approximately 4.5 to safeguard against excessive microbial growth.

The pancreas has a pH level ranging from 8.0 to 8.3.

Intestines: the pH of the small intestine ranges from 6.0 to 7.4, while the large intestine has a pH range of 5.7 to 6.7.

Blood maintains a pH level within a narrow range of 7.35 to 7.45.

Although various parts of the body have varying pH levels, the blood serves as the balance point for maintaining homeostasis in the body. Homeostasis refers to the natural inclination for a balanced and stable state to be maintained among interconnected components. The body works tirelessly to maintain a stable equilibrium by providing the necessary nutrients for organ health.

In order to achieve homeostasis in the body, it is crucial for the blood to maintain a pH level of 7.4. When the blood's pH drops below a certain level, it can lead to shock and even death due to metabolic acidosis. It is crucial to uphold this slightly alkaline state in the blood as it helps to decrease the hydrogen levels in the blood. An excess of hydrogen in the blood can lead to a decrease in hemoglobin levels in red blood cells, which can hinder the efficient transportation of oxygen and nutrients to cells in the body. This can have negative effects on the health of your organs and metabolic functions.

The body's buffering systems work to keep the pH level at a steady 7.4. The buffering systems can become overwhelmed when the body is consistently supplied with acidic foods. The body will extract alkaline material, such as calcium, from bones and fluids throughout the body in order to maintain the pH balance of the blood. This can have a negative impact on the health of organs and their metabolic functions, potentially leading to the development of chronic diseases such as osteoporosis, kidney disease, heart disease, and liver disease. Plant foods and herbs help maintain the body's pH levels, supporting overall health.

WATER

Water is frequently underestimated, yet it plays a crucial role in promoting the optimal functioning of the human genome. Many individuals following a Western diet fail to consume an adequate amount of fruits and vegetables, despite their high water content. It is generally recommended to consume one gallon of water per day, which includes water from both food and beverages. It would be wise to consume a gallon of water, allowing the body to eliminate any excess.

Spring water is the preferred choice for drinking. This product includes natural minerals that help maintain water quality and safeguard against harmful bacteria. Avoid drinking tap water. Regular tap water often contains chemicals such as chlorine and fluoride, which are added to kill bacteria and protect teeth. However, these chemicals can be harmful to the body and disrupt its natural balance.

PROTEIN

An esteemed herbalist did not prioritize the term or concept of protein as it contradicted their healing approach. He focused on minerals or elements instead. Elements such as nitrogen are essential for the growth and function of muscles and enzymes. The body depends on the absorption of nitrogen compounds to sustain essential structures like muscles and enzymes. There is a common misconception that consuming meat is necessary to obtain nitrogen compounds, but this belief is unfounded.

Plants also contain nitrogen-based compounds similar to those found in meat, known as proteins. These nitrogenous organic compounds are made up of large molecules of amino acids, which are essential building blocks for muscle, hair, collagen, enzymes, and antibodies.

Ever since a study conducted in 1914 revealed that infant rats experienced faster growth when consuming animal protein instead of vegetable protein, the meat industry has launched a powerful campaign to maintain animal protein's reign as the superior source of protein. Many people are unaware that plants contain protein and mistakenly believe that consuming meat is necessary to obtain these nitrogen compounds. The campaign's success has contributed to this misconception. This campaign has been and continues to be used to encourage the adoption of a Western diet, which has a significant correlation with the onset of chronic diseases. In addition to the campaign's achievement of causing some individuals to overlook the fact that plants contain protein, it also managed to convince many people that plant protein is an incomplete protein. Plant protein lacks the nine essential amino acids that are necessary for the body and must be obtained through consumption.

The conclusion of the 1914 study, which claimed that vegetable protein was incomplete, was later found to be incorrect. However, this finding had minimal impact. The meat industry successfully influenced health organizations to advocate for the consumption of meat protein instead of vegetable sources of nitrogen compounds. As a result, the general population came to believe that meat protein was essential for optimal growth and health. Advocates for a plant-based diet and plant-based protein, such as John McDougall, MD, were successful in maintaining pressure on these health organizations. Organizations such as the American Heart Association have come to recognize that plant protein is a complete protein, eliminating the need for protein combining to meet the daily recommended value. The organization recently made a statement on their website about the nutritional content of whole grains, legumes, vegetables, seeds, and nuts. There is no need to consciously combine these foods, known as "complimentary proteins," within a single meal. Despite being readily accessible on the website, a significant number of individuals remain uninformed about the statement, leading them to hold the misconception that vegetable protein is of lower quality.

Animal protein was considered the superior protein due to its ability to promote faster growth in infant rats. There was also a downside to this growth, which received little attention or publicity. The amino acid composition in meat protein closely resembles the amino acid makeup in the body, which is why consuming it promotes accelerated growth. Consuming it as more than 10 percent of the daily calories also contributed to the accelerated growth of cancer cells. No similar association was observed in relation to the intake of vegetable protein. The vegetable protein composition effectively promotes natural human growth while maintaining the health of cells and preventing the growth of harmful organisms.

NITROGEN SATURATED PLANT FOODS

While all plants contain complete amino acids, some plant foods have a higher concentration of nitrogen compounds than others. Grains, legumes, nuts, and seeds typically have a higher protein content compared to fruits and vegetables.

Selection of grains: Amaranth, fonio, kamut, quinoa, rye, spelt, teff, wild rice

Legumes: Garbanzo beans (chickpeas) Assortment of nuts and seeds: Brazil nuts, hemp seeds, pine nuts, raw sesame "tahini" butter, walnuts

---

MILK

Enjoy a variety of plant-based milk options like hemp-seed milk, coconut milk, and walnut milk. It is advisable to prepare your own milk to ensure the purity of the nut or seed milk you consume. Check out the recipes.

ENERGY

Fruits are packed with natural carbohydrates and serve as the body's main source of energy. Opting for fresh fruits is a healthier choice compared to canned fruits. Canned fruits undergo processing and may contain additives and preservatives that can potentially be harmful.

Apples, bananas, berries, cantaloupe, cherries, currants, dates, figs, grapes (seeded), key limes, mango, melons (seeded), oranges, papayas, peaches, pears, plums, prickly pear, prunes, raisins (seeded), soft jelly coconuts, soursops, tamarind.

CLEANSING

Vegetables provide a rich source of micronutrients such as vitamins, minerals, phytonutrients, and fiber. These nutrients nourish the body and support the health of the digestive tract, which plays a crucial role in the body's immune system.

Enjoy a variety of fresh and nutritious ingredients such as amaranth greens, avocado, bell peppers, chayote, cucumber, dandelion greens, garbanzo beans, green banana, izote, kale, lettuce, mushrooms, nopales, okra, olives, onions, purslane, poke salad, sea vegetables, squash, tomato, tomatillo, turnip greens, watercress, and zucchini.

OILS

It is advisable to limit the consumption of oils as they are not considered a whole food. Excessive oil intake can contribute to inflammation, the risk of developing diabetes, and harm to arteries.

Use grape-seed oil sparingly as it is high in omega-6. Opt for sesame oil, hempseed oil, avocado oil, and olive oil (avoid cooking with it as high heat can compromise its quality). Similarly, it's best to avoid cooking with coconut oil to preserve its integrity.

SEASONINGS

Ingredients include achiote, basil, bay leaf, cayenne (African bird pepper), cilantro, coriander, dill, habanero, onion powder, oregano, powdered granulated seaweed (kelp, dulce, nori), pure sea salt, sage, savory, sweet basil, tarragon, and thyme.

HERBAL TEAS

Choosing herbal teas over regular teas, such as green tea, is a wise choice. Not only do herbal teas lack caffeine, but they also offer a diverse array of phytonutrients that can boost the immune system.

Alvaca, anise, chamomile, cloves, fennel, ginger, lemongrass, red raspberry, and sea-moss tea

---

SUGARS

Just like with oils, it's best to limit your intake of added sugar. Date Sugar is the optimal choice for consumption from a health perspective. Date sugar is made by drying and grinding dates. The nutrients remain intact, with the exception of water, which helps regulate the digestion of sugar.

Agave syrup made from pure cactus is excellent, although the way it is processed may affect its carbohydrate structure. (Grade B maple syrup and maple sugar are no longer included in the recommended food list. Certain manufacturers of maple syrup and sugar sometimes utilize formaldehyde to maintain the opening in the maple tree for sap extraction. Formaldehyde is a hazardous substance that can contaminate the sap and pose health risks.

CHAPTER 3

PREPARING HERBS

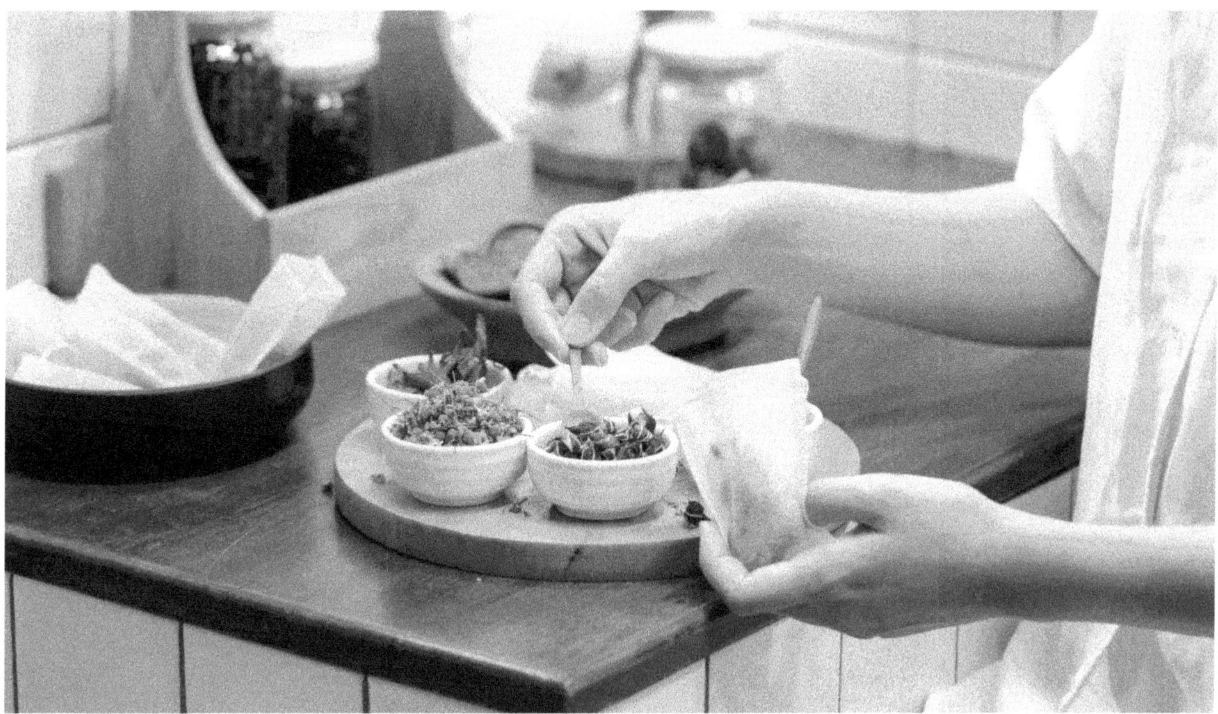

Consider medicinal herbs as plants with enhanced strength. Medicinal herbs contain a wealth of nutrients and phytonutrients, which are beneficial chemical components. They are commonly utilized to combat diseases and for occasional detoxification. Herbs are most effective when paired with alkaline plant foods. When consuming medicinal herbs, it is important to avoid certain foods such as meat, dairy, processed foods, and acidic plant foods. These foods can reduce the effectiveness of the herbs' chemical components. Consuming these foods can introduce harmful substances that disrupt the body's natural balance and impair the functioning of organs and metabolic processes.

Understanding the most effective herbs for treating specific diseases is crucial when using herbal remedies to combat illness. Another factor to consider is whether you prefer commercially encapsulated or tonic herbs, or if you prefer to prepare your own herbs using whole herbs that you either grow yourself or buy in bulk. Opting for encapsulated or tonic herbs is a convenient choice, as it eliminates the need for any preparation and provides clear dosages on the packaging. Simply familiarize yourself with the herbs to purchase. While opting for this mode, there is a higher risk of the herbs not being genuine or of inferior quality. It is widely recognized that herbal supplements have undergone testing, revealing that the contents of the package often do not match what is advertised. It can be challenging to identify the specific herbs you are purchasing since encapsulated herbs are ground into a powder, making it hard to differentiate between them.

If you have the opportunity to cultivate your own herbs, it's advisable to obtain seeds from plants that have been gathered from the wild or transplant wildcrafted plants to your growing area. It's best to cultivate them under conditions that closely mimic their natural environment, avoiding the use of synthetic fertilizers. Wildcrafted plants are plants that grow freely in their natural environment, untouched by human hands. The plants thrive under unique conditions that enhance their natural vitality and promote the development of their nutrients and phytonutrients to their highest potential. To ensure the best possible growth for these plants in a controlled growing environment, it is essential to utilize the natural fertilizer that nature offers.

I have discovered that an effective method for enriching the soil and promoting robust plant growth is to collect organic waste, such as leftover plant parts and plant-based meals.

Grind them thoroughly with water and utilize this as a fertilizer. By recycling plant foods, you can effectively return unused minerals back to the soil. This is the natural process, without any artificial intervention. The leaves and fruits naturally fall to the ground and are recycled by being absorbed back into the soil, creating a cycle of restoration. If you're unable to cultivate your own herbs, a great alternative is to purchase whole herbs in large quantities.

HARVESTING MEDICINAL HERBS

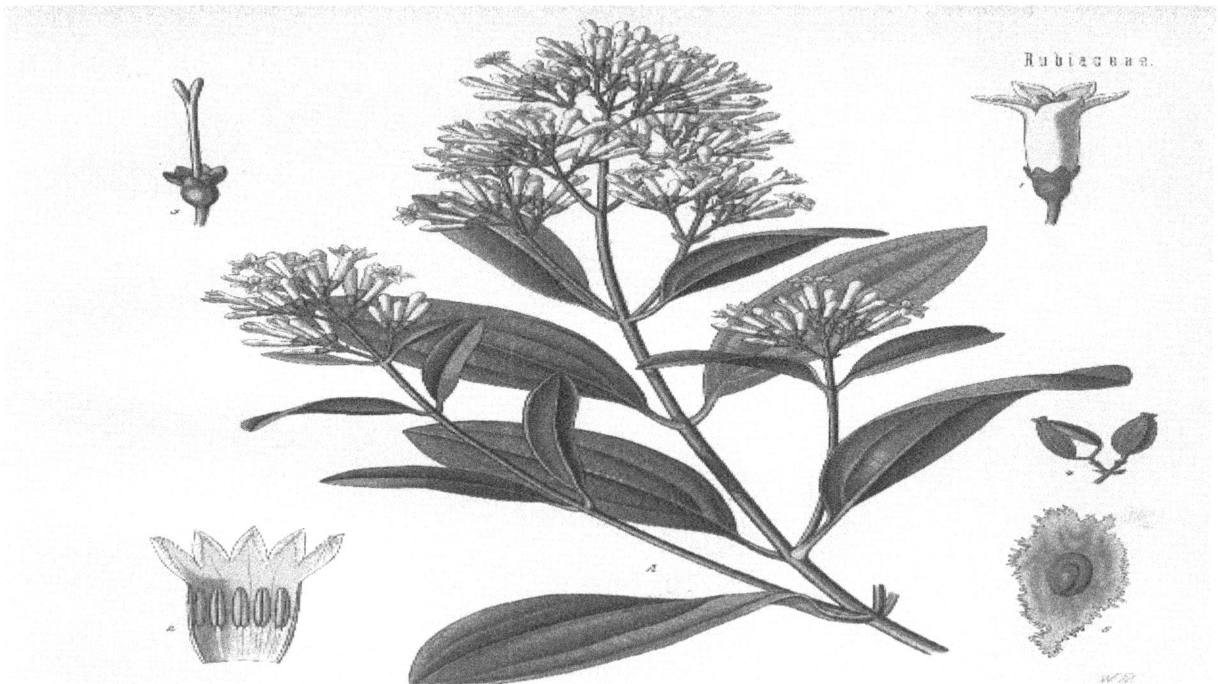

Roots, leaves, buds, and flowers are typically harvested at different times to ensure that each part is picked at its peak of energy and vitality.

ROOTS

Typically, the optimal time to gather medicinal roots is during the early spring or fall, when the roots contain a higher concentration of the plant's energy. In the spring and summer months, the energy and nutrients stored in the roots are transported to the leaves and flowers. During the fall season, energy and nutrients are stored in the roots to nourish the leaves and flowers in the upcoming spring.

LEAVES

Leaves are typically harvested prior to the plant's flowering or seed production stage. This allows the plant to conserve energy and nutrients for the growth of leaves, rather than diverting them towards the development of flowers and fruits. Select mature leaves that are robust, display a lively hue, and show minimal to no signs of insect damage.

FLOWERS

Make sure to harvest flowers when they are just starting to open. By this stage, the flower has accumulated ample energy and nutrients, but their levels gradually diminish once the flower fully blossoms.

DRYING HERBS

If you don't plan on using the medicinal herbs immediately after harvesting, it is advisable to dry them in order to preserve their quality and nutritional value.

Conventional techniques for drying herbs involve creating compact bundles of the herbs and suspending them from a clothesline, ensuring there is ample space between each bundle to facilitate proper airflow and the drying process. It is important to ensure that the drying area for herbs is not humid. This will prevent the water from being retained in the plants instead of being drawn out. It is important to keep the area shaded to prevent any chemical reactions that could affect the quality of the herbs.

Instead of hanging the herbs from a clothesline, another option is to lay them out on a screen, ensuring they are spaced apart to allow for optimal airflow. It is recommended to hang or elevate the screens to promote proper airflow.

Another option is to use a dehydrator to dry the herbs, which will speed up the drying process. It is crucial to maintain a specific temperature range of 90° to 105°F in order to preserve the integrity of the nutrients and phytonutrients.

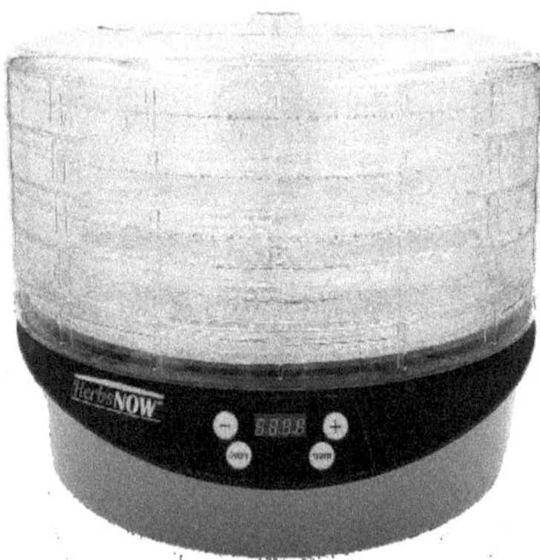

Once the herbs have dried, it's important to store them in glass jars with lids that seal tightly to maintain their freshness. Properly ventilating the herbs will gradually diminish the potency of their components. To ensure the herbs maintain their medicinal potency for an extended period, it is recommended to store them in a cool, dark, and dry place.

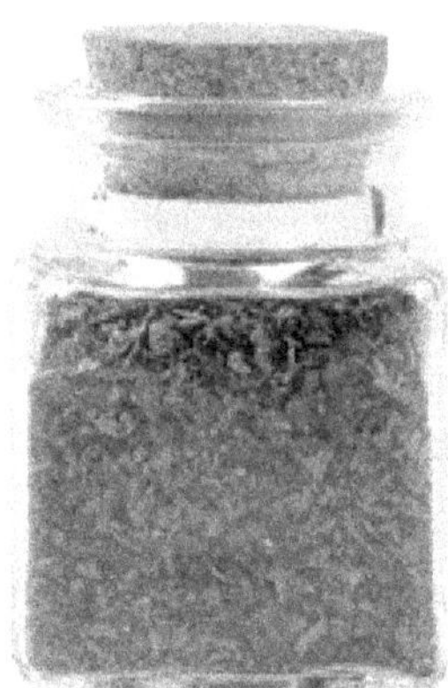

Instead of harvesting your own herbs, you have the option to buy whole herbs in bulk. This would be a superior choice compared to buying prepackaged encapsulated herbs, although the capsules are the most convenient to use. Purchasing herbs in bulk allows for a more thorough examination of the product, ensuring its authenticity and quality. You can make comparisons to what you have observed or to visual representations.

Bulk herb packages typically contain whole herbs, although occasionally they may contain ground or powdered herbs. For optimal quality control, it is recommended to purchase whole herbs or herb pieces and grind them into a fine powder. When you're prepared to utilize a portion of the herb, simply grind it down. You have the option to enclose the herbs within vegetable capsules and keep them in a container. For optimal storage, it is recommended to place the ground herb in a glass jar with a secure lid to maintain freshness. For optimal preservation of the medicinal compounds in the herbs, it is advisable to store them in a cool, dark, and dry environment.

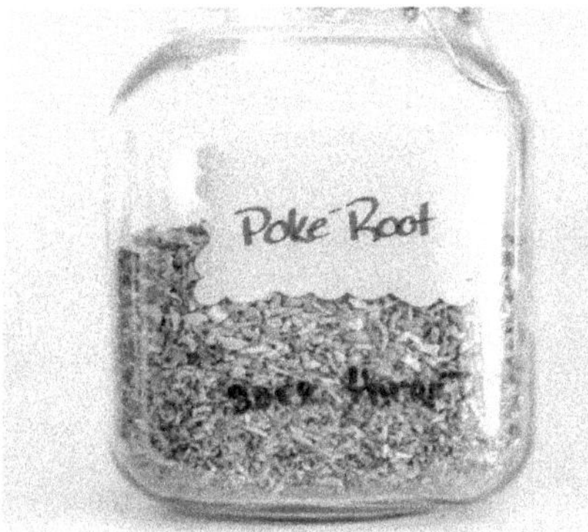

Herbal distributors often offer bulk herbs in sixteen-ounce packages. You can also find herbs in larger and smaller packages, depending on your preference. Most bulk herbs are typically sold as whole pieces, although there are a few that are available in powdered form.

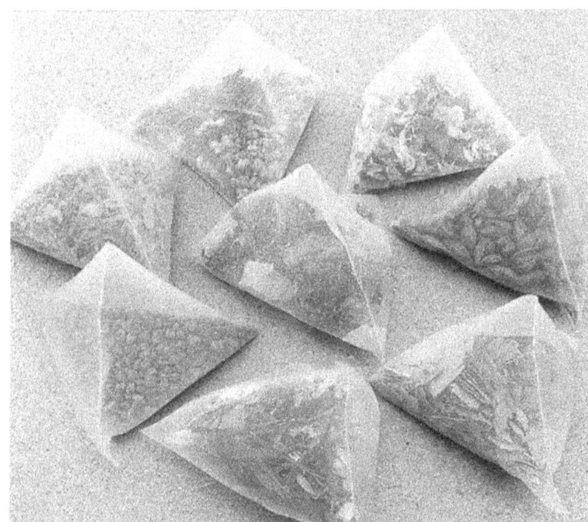

MAKING HERBS

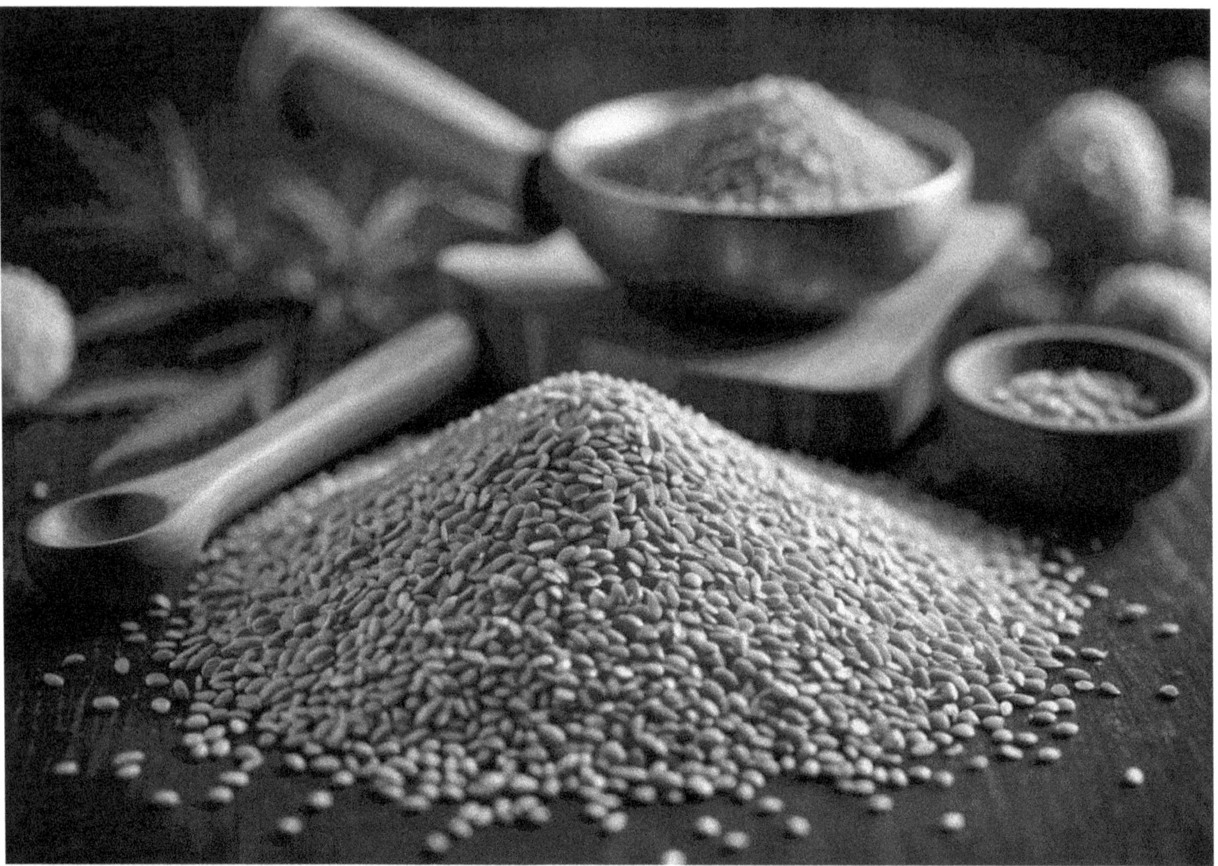

There are different ways to create medicinal herbs, such as breaking down whole herbs into smaller parts or using extraction methods to remove chemical compounds from the herbs. I usually opt for using the entire herb, either by grinding it down and encapsulating it or by drinking it with water. This way, I can make the most of all the fiber and components that are naturally present. The extraction method is utilized to efficiently introduce the chemical components into the bloodstream, bypassing the need for the body to break down the herbs and extract the chemical compounds from the fiber. There are both advantages and disadvantages to this. Utilizing medicinal herbs in this manner can effectively saturate the bloodstream with chemical components, although it may be slightly excessive.

The kidneys diligently maintain the delicate balance of minerals, water, and other compounds. When there is an influx of chemical components in the bloodstream, the kidneys are compelled to eliminate some of them by passing them to the bladder and ultimately out of the body. On the other hand, when the herbs are ground down into finer particles, the body can access a greater amount of the herbs' chemicals in a more regulated manner.

It is advisable to avoid consuming large pieces of herbs, as the intact plant cell walls are resistant to being broken down. The chemical compounds of the herbs are contained within the cell walls of the leaf, flower, root, bark, or seed. Thoroughly chewing your food is crucial for maximizing nutrient absorption into the bloodstream. Consuming large or whole pieces of herbs can hinder the release and absorption of nutrients.

It can be quite challenging to effectively chew raw plant materials like leaves, flowers, roots, bark, and seeds in order to fully break down their cell walls and release the majority of their nutrients.

When herbs are ground into smaller particles, the digestive process can access a greater amount of the herbs' compounds more efficiently.

By ensuring the proper balance of fiber and compounds, digestion is regulated, preventing an excessive influx of nutrients into the bloodstream and maintaining the optimal levels of minerals and components. Grinding herbs allows for quicker digestion and absorption of nutrients into the bloodstream compared to consuming whole herbs in large portions. This enhances the efficiency of the herbs' digestion, unlike ingesting the extracted compounds from herbs, allowing the body to make better use of the nutrients.

For certain herbs or routine maintenance, infusions or decoctions can be a better choice for medicinal herb extractions.

INFUSION

Infusions are made by steeping leaves, buds, flowers, berries, and some seeds of plants in boiling water to extract their medicinal properties.

Infusions are crafted using the delicate components of plants, as immersing them in hot water is sufficient to effectively permeate the herb's cellular structure. By infusing the softer parts of the plants, a significant amount of the herb's components can be released into the water.

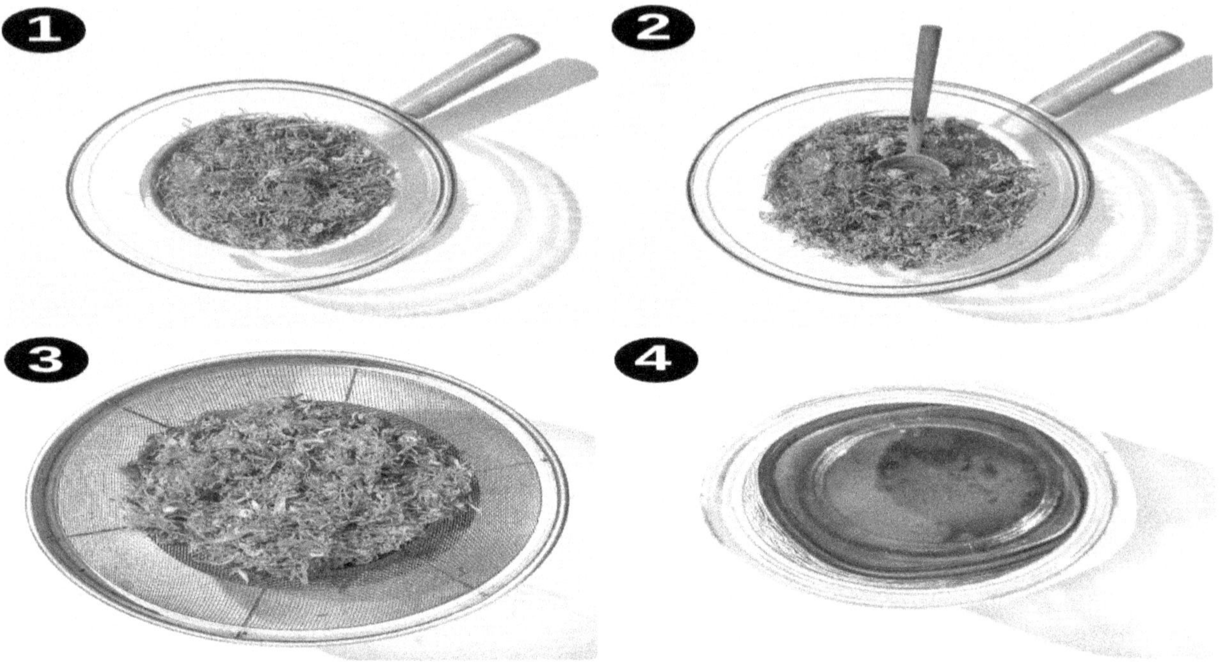

Preparation

Step 1: Use either 1 tablespoon of dried herb or 1½ tablespoons of fresh herb.

Step 2: Bring 8 ounces to a boil and then remove from heat.

Step 3: Include the herb in the water. Allow to steep for 30 to 45 minutes. The longer you allow the herb to steep, the greater the extraction of chemical components as the water remains hot. The intensity of the infusion increases as the water takes on a deeper or more vibrant hue, indicating the release of more components from the herb.

Step 4: Filter the infusion and enjoy.

Increase the amount of infusion by multiplying the measurement of herb and water by the same number. If you use 4 tablespoons of herb, you would need to use 32 ounces of water.

DECOCTION

Decoctions are similar to infusions, as they utilize the hardier components of the plant such as roots, twigs, and bark. Given the nature of these plant parts, pouring boiling water on them will only result in a minimal release of the herb's components. Boiling and simmering these parts of the plant helps to efficiently extract their chemicals.

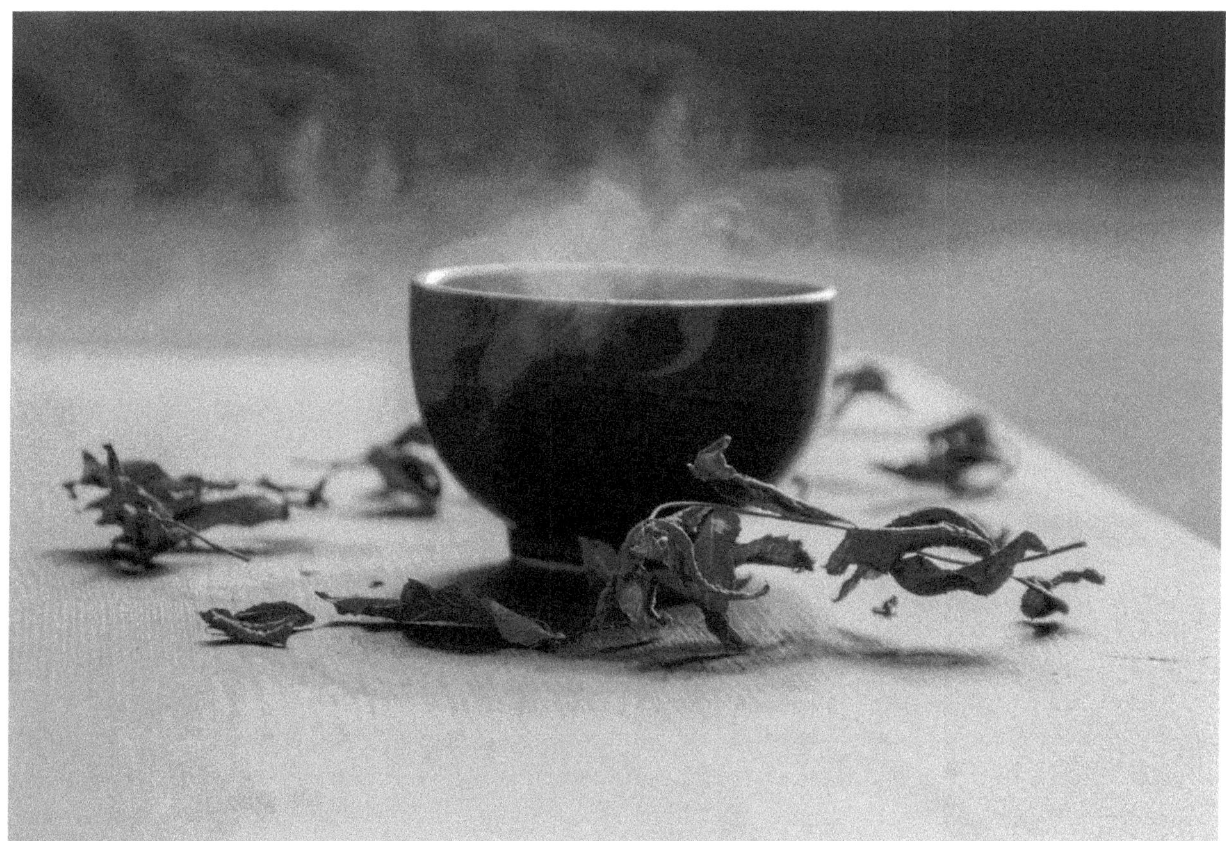

Preparation

Step 1: Use either 1 tablespoon of dried herb or 1½ tablespoons of fresh herb.

Step 2: Add 8 ounces of water and herb to a saucepan.

Step 3: Heat the water in a covered pot until it reaches boiling point, then lower the heat and let it simmer on a low setting for 30 minutes. The duration of simmering the water directly affects the concentration of components extracted.

Step 4: Allow the water to cool before transferring the mixture into a mason jar.

Follow the instructions carefully to enhance the potency of the decoction

GRINDING HERBS, ENCAPSULATION, AND DOSAGE

GRINDING

For optimal results, it is recommended to consume the herb in its ground whole form. To ensure optimal digestion, a regular coffee grinder can effectively grind the delicate parts of plants such as leaves, buds, flowers, and certain seeds into finer particles.

For tougher materials such as twigs, branches, roots, and bark, an industrial grinder or a heavy-duty industrial blender is required. Industrial grinders will have enhanced capabilities to effortlessly grind the toughest parts of the plants into a fine powder.

Industrial blenders are capable of grinding down the tougher parts of plants, although it may take a bit more time. However, they are more efficient at grinding herbs into less fine particles.

ENCAPSULATION

You can purchase affordable encapsulation kits that simplify the process of encapsulating herbs. Cap M Quik offers kits for different capsule sizes, including "0", "00", and "000". I use a "00" kit with vegetarian capsules. The capsules are filled with approximately 500 mg of herb.

DOSAGE

The typical dosages for herbs are calculated for an average adult weighing approximately 150 pounds.

For an adult weighing around 150 pounds, the maximum recommended dosage of a herbal extract is six grams per day. This dosage is commonly used for the entire herbs as well, although herbal extracts contain higher concentrations of chemical compounds. The herb dosage per capsule is approximately 500 milligrams or 0.5 grams. In order to achieve the desired effects, it is recommended to consume a maximum of twelve capsules per day of the herb in question, each containing approximately five hundred milligrams.

The importance of precise dosage is typically higher for pharmaceutical medicine compared to herbal medicine, and for valid reasons. Approximately half of pharmaceutical medicines are sourced from plants, with the distinction being that pharmaceutical medicine extracts the active compound from a plant and either concentrates it or replicates it synthetically. The concentration of the active ingredient is significantly stronger and poses a greater risk compared to herbal medicine. This is due to the unusually high amount of the active ingredient entering the body and the absence of other plant nutrients that would typically regulate its digestion. Even though the pharmaceutical medicine is derived from a natural source, it does not have the same impact on the body as natural remedies. Herbal medicine is generally more lenient, but it is still important to avoid intentionally consuming excessive amounts of herbs. Excessive amounts of anything can disrupt the body's natural processes.

Typically, the recommended dosages for herbs on commercial bottled herbal products are usually two or three capsules, taken two or three times a day. Capsules typically contain approximately 500 milligrams of herb, allowing for a maximum daily dosage of nine capsules, which would amount to 4500 mg or 4.5 g per day.

This dosage is still significantly lower than what is recommended. If you prefer loose herbs over capsules, the amount equivalent to one capsule is roughly a quarter teaspoon. Taking two or three capsules a day is equivalent to consuming a moderate amount of the herb. It is recommended to take this dosage two or three times daily, with a maximum daily intake of just over two teaspoons.

In herbal medicine, herbs are commonly combined to address specific conditions, cleanse organs, or support specific functions. Although this dosage is for a single herb, it is important to consider the potential benefits of combining herbs. Various herbs contain distinct chemical compounds that target the same condition or situation using unique approaches. Even though the chemical compounds vary, the dosages are typically decreased for each herb to ensure they stay within the recommended daily limit of six grams per day, or a maximum of nine daily commercial herbal capsules.

This information aims to provide a comprehensive understanding of how herbs and dosages are prepared, for educational purposes. While some individuals may utilize this information to enhance their knowledge of herb preparation, it is crucial to recognize that herbalists devote significant time to studying herbs and their medicinal preparation. As a result, they possess a deeper understanding of the intricate details involved in the process.

Herbalists will gain a deeper understanding of how to combine herbs and adjust their dosage.

If you were combining herbs and each one used the same dosage, then determining the dose for the combined herbs would be quite simple.

Mixing together a combination of different herbs is essential. One option is to package the mixed herbs according to the recommended dosages found in commercial herbal products. Alternatively, you can measure out the equivalent amount of loose herb and consume it with water or a vegetable or fruit smoothie.

It's important to understand the proper way to combine herbs to maximize their effectiveness and avoid using too little of a specific herb.

It is generally advised to limit the number of herbs to four or five when combining them to target a specific issue. Using more herbs may require adjusting the dosage accordingly. A seasoned herbalist would be better equipped to make an informed decision regarding the dosage adjustment in this situation. Adding to the complexity is the fact that certain herbs are used in smaller amounts than the usual recommended dosage. This further complicates the process of combining herbs and determining the appropriate dose for each one.

CHAPTER 4

ALKALINE MEDICINAL HERBS

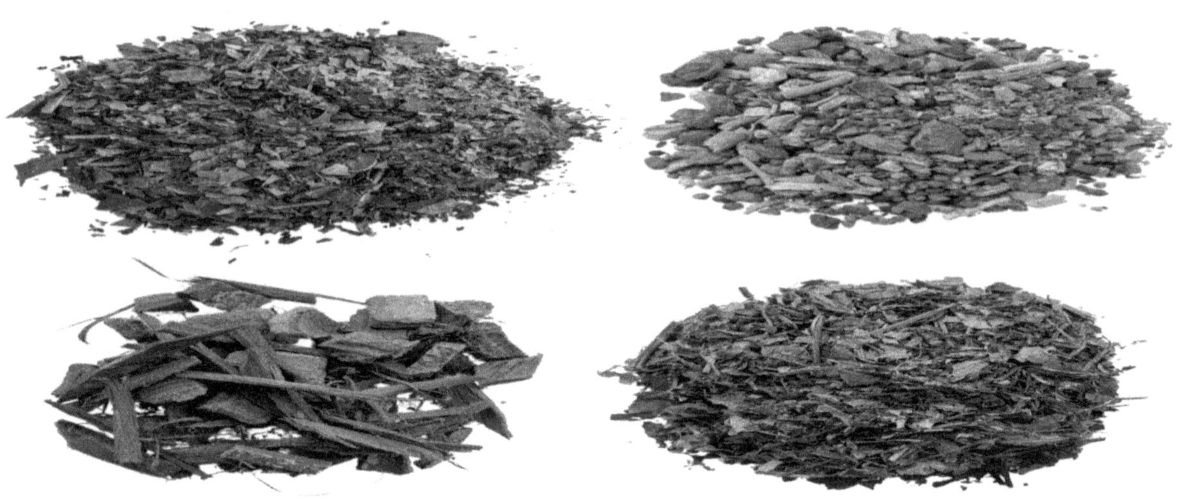

The alkaline movement is growing in popularity, thanks to the efforts of a well-known herbalist who has been instrumental in promoting the African Bio Mineral Balance. Many herbalists rely on a diverse selection of herbs to successfully address and reverse various illnesses. This individual has been instrumental in identifying the natural alkaline herbs that have proven to be beneficial for the overall health of the African genome, which is applicable to everyone.

These herbs are of the highest quality, with their chemical composition remaining pure and untouched by any form of alteration. Herbs that have predominantly thrived in African environments or similar conditions, sharing a genetic affinity with the African genome, exhibit a chemical connection. These herbs contribute to creating a harmonious atmosphere within the body, fostering stability and rejuvenation on physical, mental, emotional, and spiritual levels for everyone. These herbs are essential for promoting healing and reversing disease.

While this herbalist's list of herbs that are beneficial for the African genome may not include every option, these herbs stand out from other commonly used herbs that are often hybrid and acidic in nature. While these other herbs do offer some benefits, they also introduce compounds that do not interact well with the body, disrupt its balance, and decrease the effectiveness of the herb. Herbs such as comfrey and the well-known echinacea are included in this category due to their incomplete chemical structure resulting from hybridization, genetic modifications, or biological manipulation.

I will discuss the alkaline herbs that this herbalist utilizes to combat disease, which have a long history in traditional medicine, spanning centuries if not millennia. I would also like to mention some herbs that may not be included in this herbalist's list but are native to regions with a climate similar to Africa, such as the guinea hen weed of Jamaica..

HERBS AND THEIR PROPERTIES

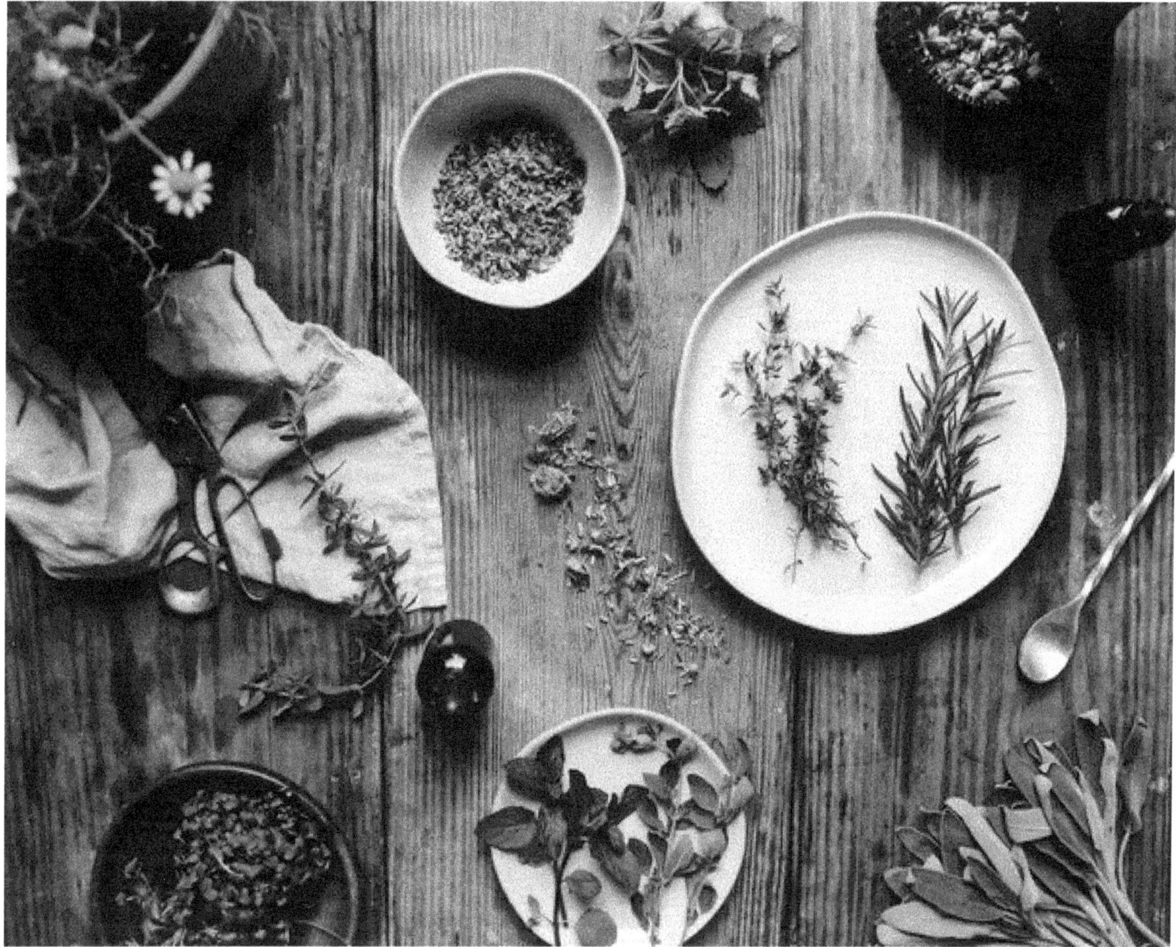

Strictly for educational purposes only. This information has not been reviewed by the appropriate regulatory authority. This information is provided for informational purposes only and should not be used as a substitute for professional medical advice. It is always recommended to consult with a healthcare professional before making any changes to your health routine. The dosages provided are for individual herbs, while the dosages for herbal combinations are discussed in the following chapter.

Arnica

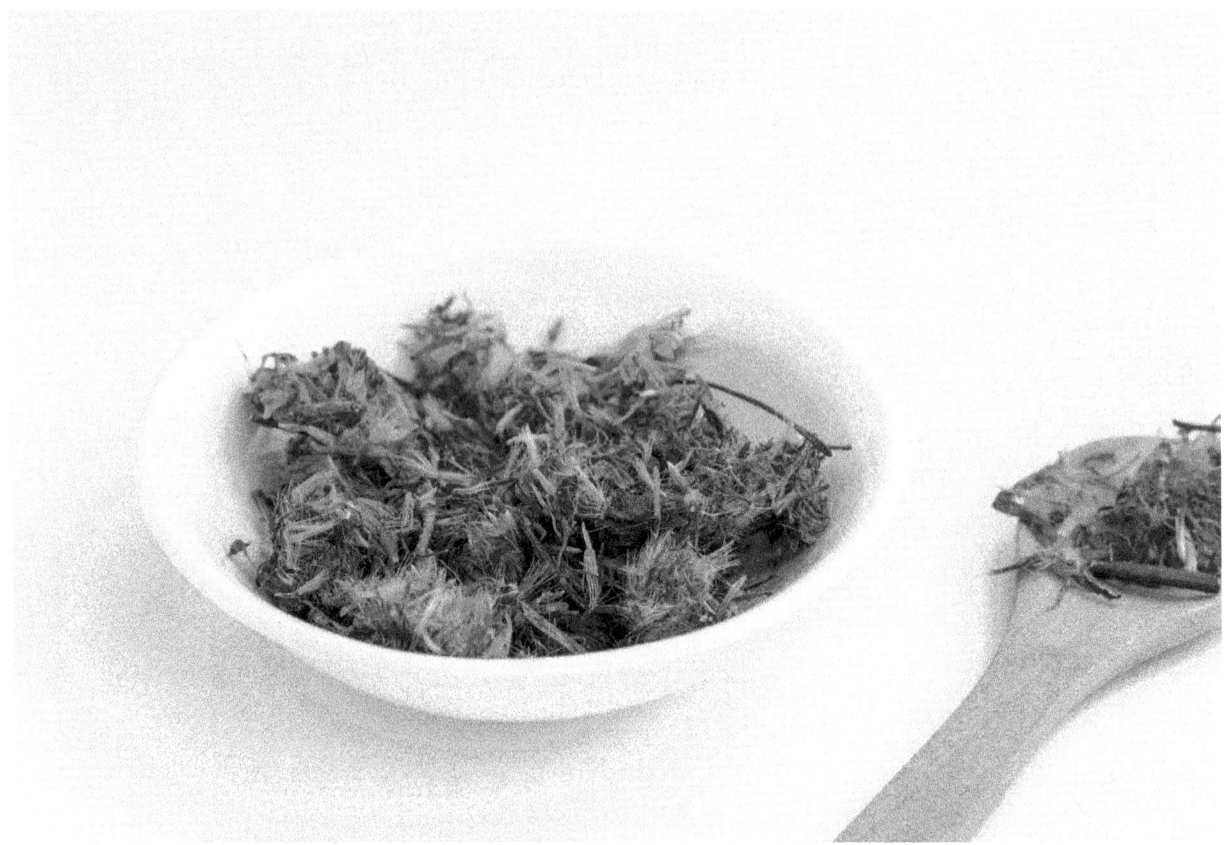

Arnica, also known as Arnica montana, Radix Ptarmicae Montanae, arnica flowers, or mountain tobacco, is a potent herb with strong anti-inflammatory and antiseptic properties. It is commonly used to address external injuries, providing pain relief and supporting the healing process of tissues.

Topical application of Arnica is often used to relieve symptoms of arthritis, sprains, bruises, and headaches. Arnica infusions are often utilized for their antiseptic properties in the management of wounds, abscesses, and boils. Arnica is a component of a well-known herbalist's uterine wash compound.

Origin: North America

General commercial dose: Arnica is used primarily as a topical cream.

Batana

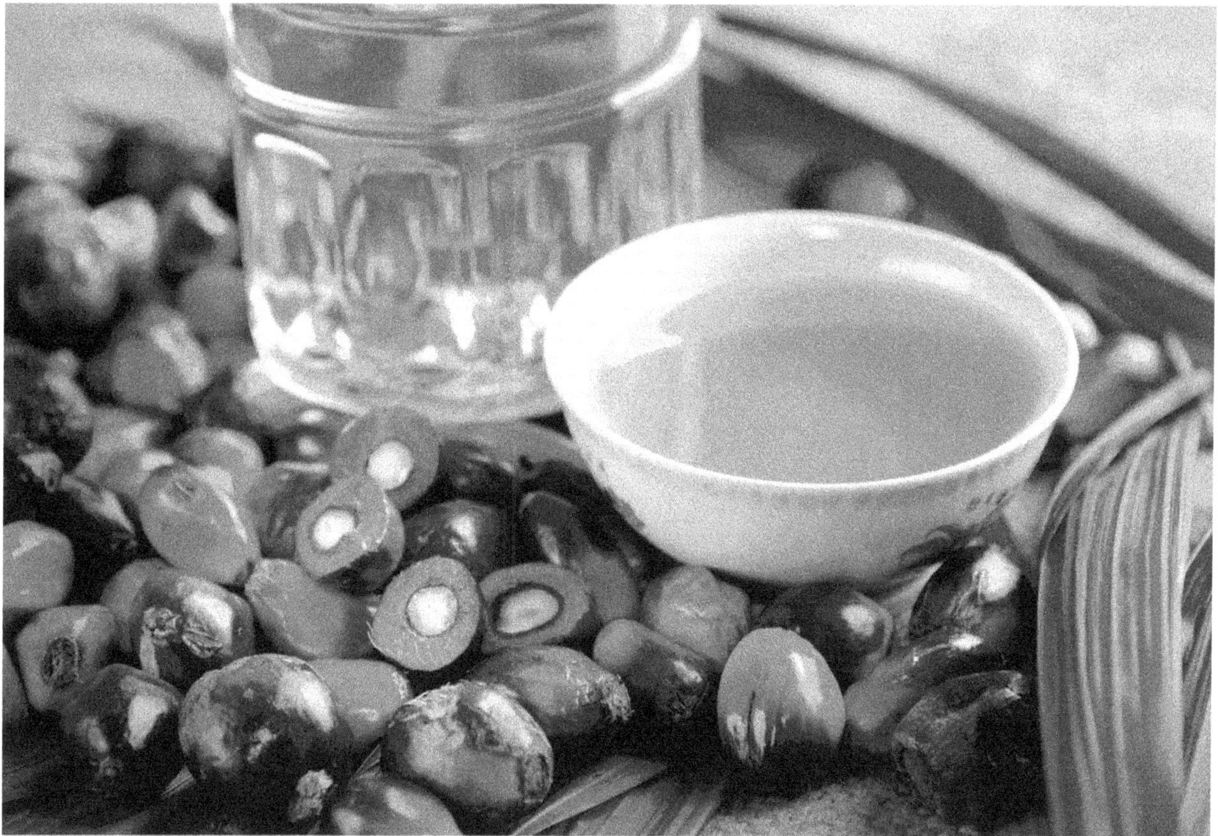

The oil is derived from the kernel of the fruit of the Elaeis oleifera tree. This oil is highly valued for its rich fatty acids, nourishing nutrients, and beneficial phytonutrients. It is commonly used as a hair oil to enhance hair strength, stimulate growth, and provide a natural coloring effect. It has the ability to naturally transform gray hair into a rich brown shade.

Origin: Honduras, Central and South America

Bladderwrack

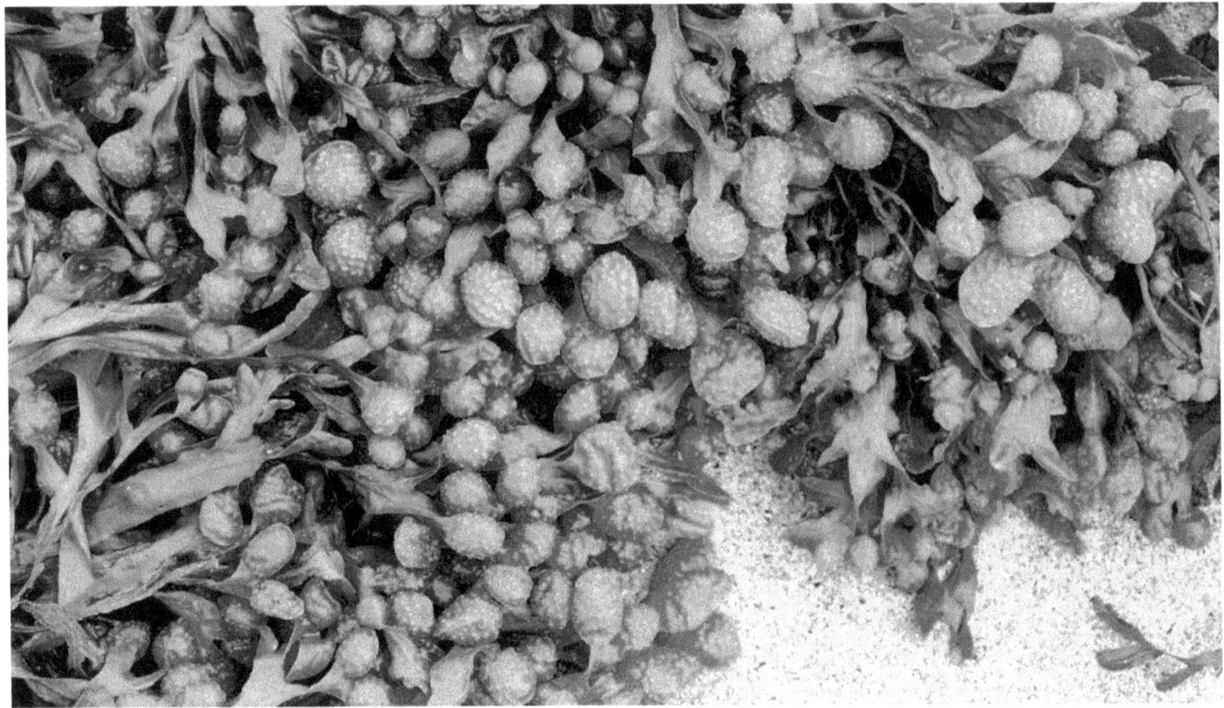

Bladderwrack (Fucus vesiculosus, fucus) is valued for its abundant iodine content. Bladderwrack has a long history of being used to address an underactive and oversized thyroid, as well as iodine deficiency. Bladderwrack is abundant in calcium, magnesium, potassium, and various other trace minerals. Bladderwrack is packed with a variety of phytonutrients that contribute to its numerous health benefits. Fucoxanthin provides a strong foundation for its antioxidant benefits.

Bladderwrack exhibits antiestrogenic properties and has demonstrated a potential to reduce the likelihood of estrogen-dependent illnesses.

Bladderwrack is effective in reducing lipid and cholesterol levels, making it beneficial for weight loss. The mucopolysaccharide phytonutrients have the ability to inhibit the enzymes responsible for breaking down the skin, resulting in reduced skin thickness and improved elasticity. Bladderwrack has also demonstrated properties that inhibit candida, bacteria, and tumor growth.

Bladderwrack is commonly used as a natural source of iodine, with each 580 mg capsule providing approximately 155 percent of the recommended daily value of iodine. It's fascinating to note that the Japanese consume 1000–3000 mcg of iodine per day without experiencing any adverse effects.

Origin: Atlantic Ocean, Pacific Ocean, North Sea, Baltic Sea

General commercial dose: One 580 mg capsule General dosage: One capsule daily

Blessed Thistle

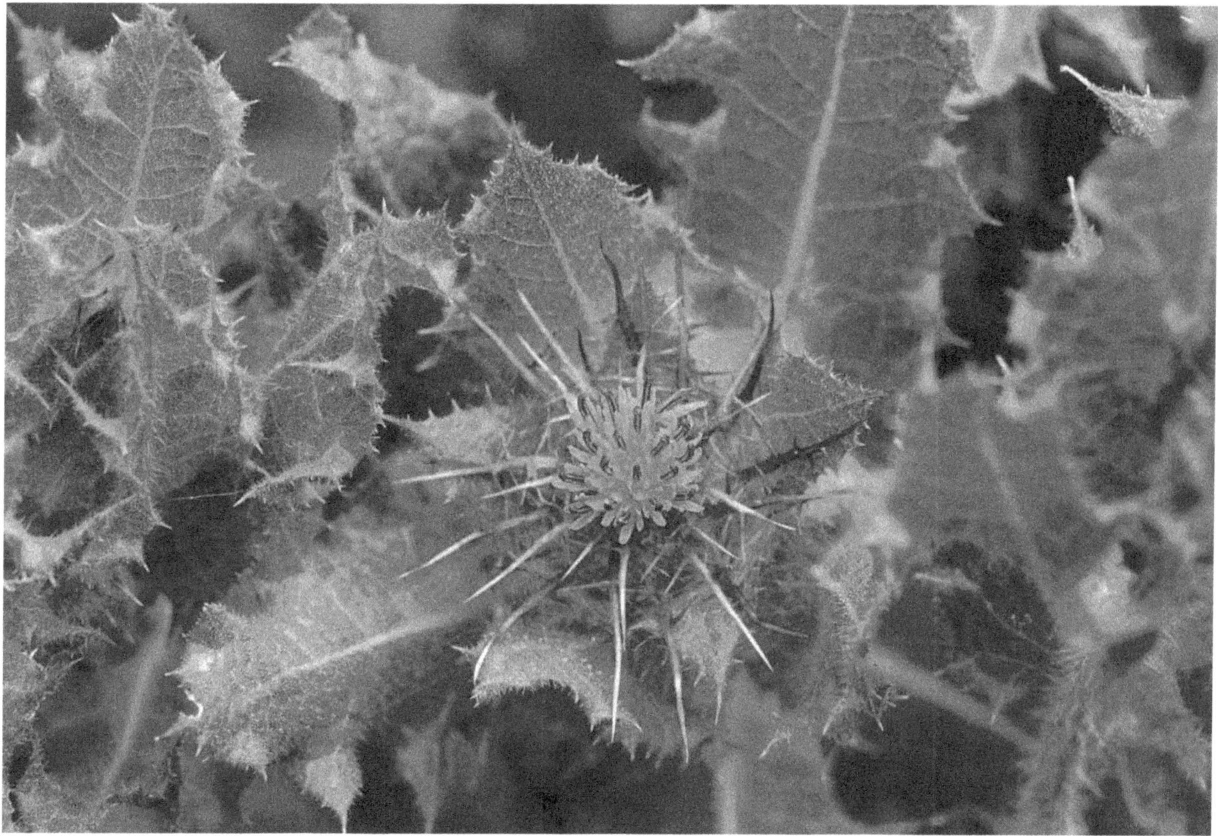

Blessed thistle, also known as Cnicus benedictus, cardo santo, centaurea benedicta, folia cardui benedicti, or holy thistle, is a member of the Asteraceae plant family. Blessed thistle is known for its high iron content and has been utilized in traditional medicine to enhance circulation and promote oxygen delivery to the brain. It is believed to aid in maintaining optimal brain function, as well as supporting the health of the heart and lungs. The bitter phytonutrients in this product are known for their ability to support liver and gallbladder function, as well as stimulate the upper digestive tract to enhance digestion and increase appetite.

Blessed thistle possesses antifungal and diuretic properties and has a long history of traditional use in treating hormonal disorders that can disrupt the menstrual cycle. Blessed thistle is also known for its ability to support lactation and enhance milk production in breastfeeding mothers. Blessed thistle is also utilized for the purpose of eliminating toxins, acids, and mucus, as well as aiding in intracellular cleansing (inside cells).

Origin: Mediterranean

General commercial dose: One 390mg capsule General dosage: Two capsules three times daily

Blue Vervain

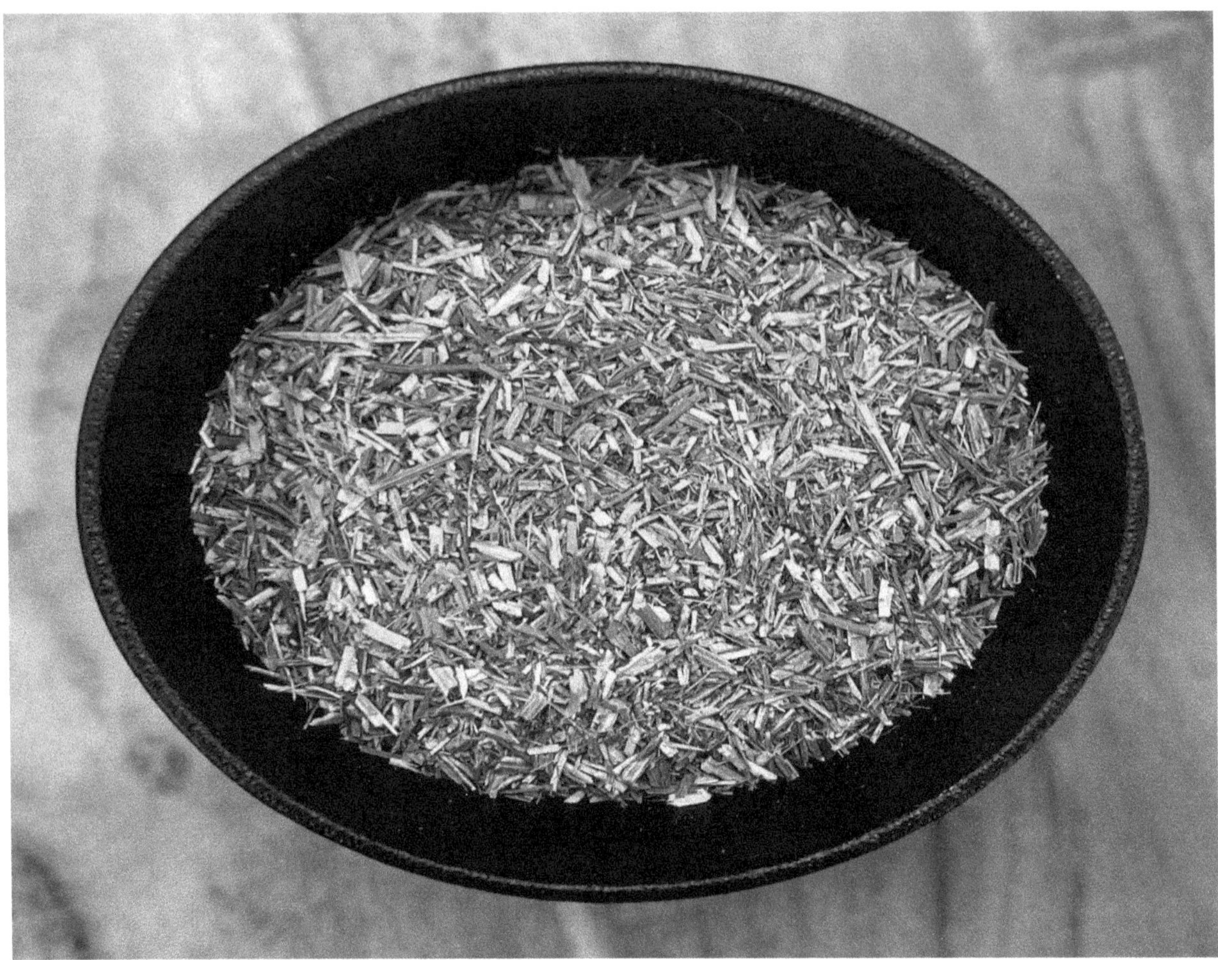

Blue vervain, also known as Verbena hastate or simpler's joy, possesses diuretic, antimalarial, anti-inflammatory, and antimicrobial properties. Blue vervain has a long history of use in traditional medicine. It has been utilized as a female tonic to alleviate menstrual cramps and as an emmenagogue to promote milk production in breastfeeding women. Blue vervain is commonly used to address nervous disorders such as stress, anxiety, and restlessness.

Origin: North America Standard commercial dose: One 400 mg capsule

Recommended dosage: Take one capsule twice a day

Burdock Root

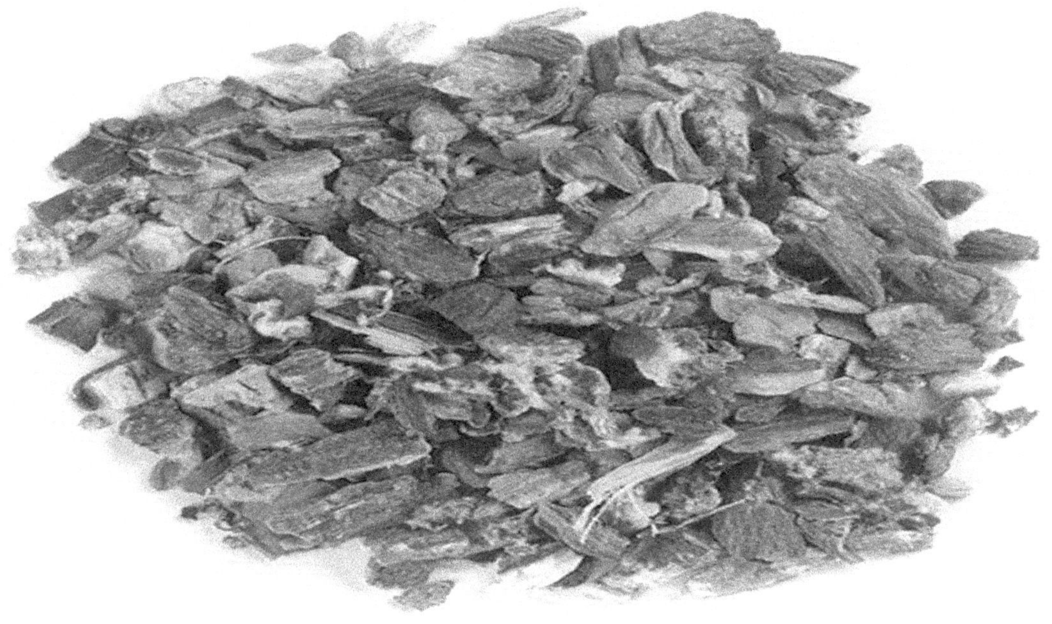

Burdock root, also referred to as bardana, is a well-known plant. Burdock root possesses a wide range of beneficial properties, including diuretic, blood cleansing, anti-inflammatory, antioxidant, antifungal, anticancer, antiviral, and antibacterial effects. Burdock root possesses a diverse range of chemical compounds, such as inulin, mucilage, essential oil, volatile oil, alkaloids, glycosides, resin, and tannins, which contribute to its numerous medicinal properties. Burdock has a long history in traditional medicine for its effectiveness in treating various skin conditions like eczema, acne, and psoriasis. It is known to aid in the elimination of toxins from the skin, promoting overall skin health. Additionally, it acts as a diuretic to encourage urination and enhance kidney function and repair. Burdock root is commonly used to purify the blood and promote liver health and function.

Origin: Africa, Asia, Europe General commercial dose: One 500 mg capsule

General dosage: Two capsules three times daily

Cascara Sagrada

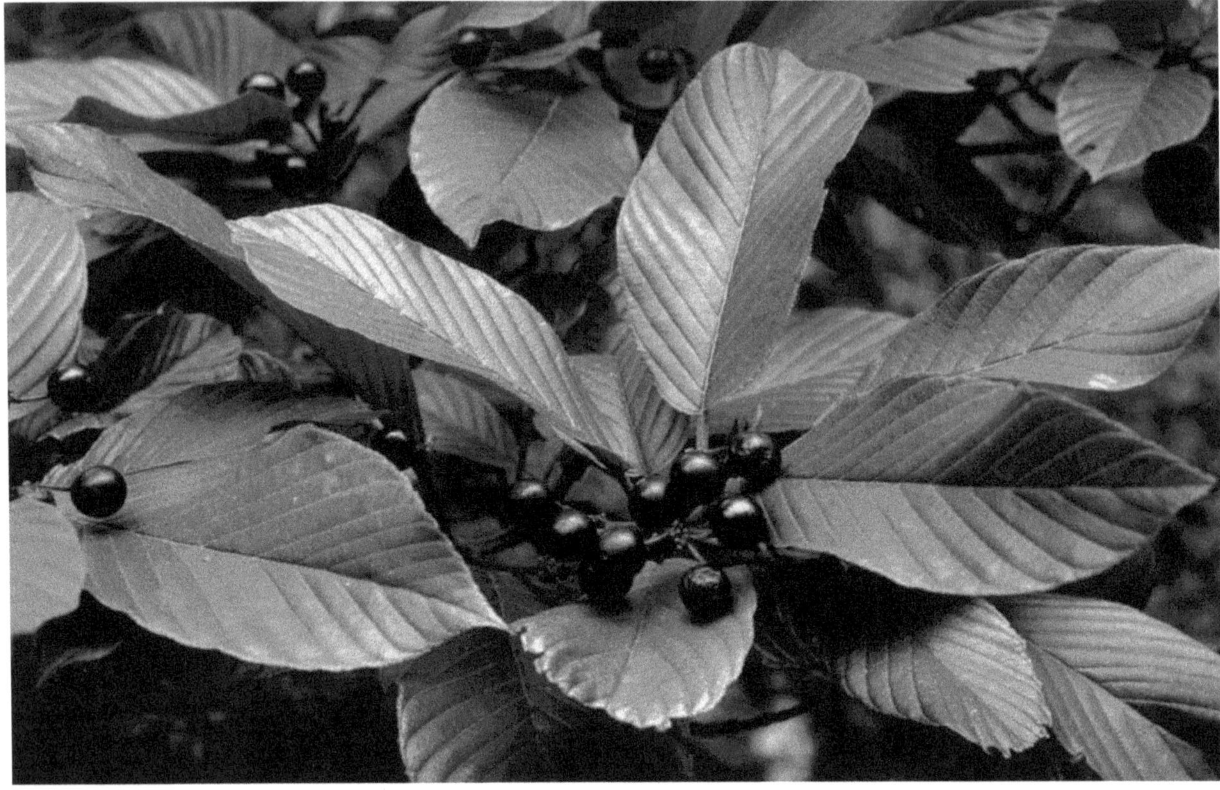

Cascara sagrada, also known as sacred bark, is rich in emodin, a compound that possesses powerful antiviral and anticancer properties. Cascara sagrada is commonly used as a laxative and helps to stimulate the natural movement of the intestines. This rhythmic movement propels waste through the intestine. This property assists in restoring the intestinal tone and promoting its overall health by facilitating the elimination of waste from pouches that form in the intestinal wall. This aids in the restoration of the mucous lining and overall health of the intestine. Cascara sagrada has a long history in traditional medicine for its potential benefits in enhancing stomach, liver, and pancreas secretions, as well as aiding in the elimination of gallstones from the gallbladder.

Origin: Western North America

General commercial dose: One 450 mg capsule General dosage: One or two capsules, preferably at bedtime

(Medical caution: Avoid usage if experiencing diarrhea or abdominal pain. It is recommended that women who are pregnant or nursing should avoid using cascara sagrada as it may stimulate labor. Additionally, lactating women should be cautious as the compound can be passed on through breastfeeding. It is not advisable to use for more than seven consecutive days. It is crucial to adhere to the recommended doses in order to prevent any potential harm to the liver. Using cascara sagrada has been proven to be safe and beneficial when used as directed.

Chaparral

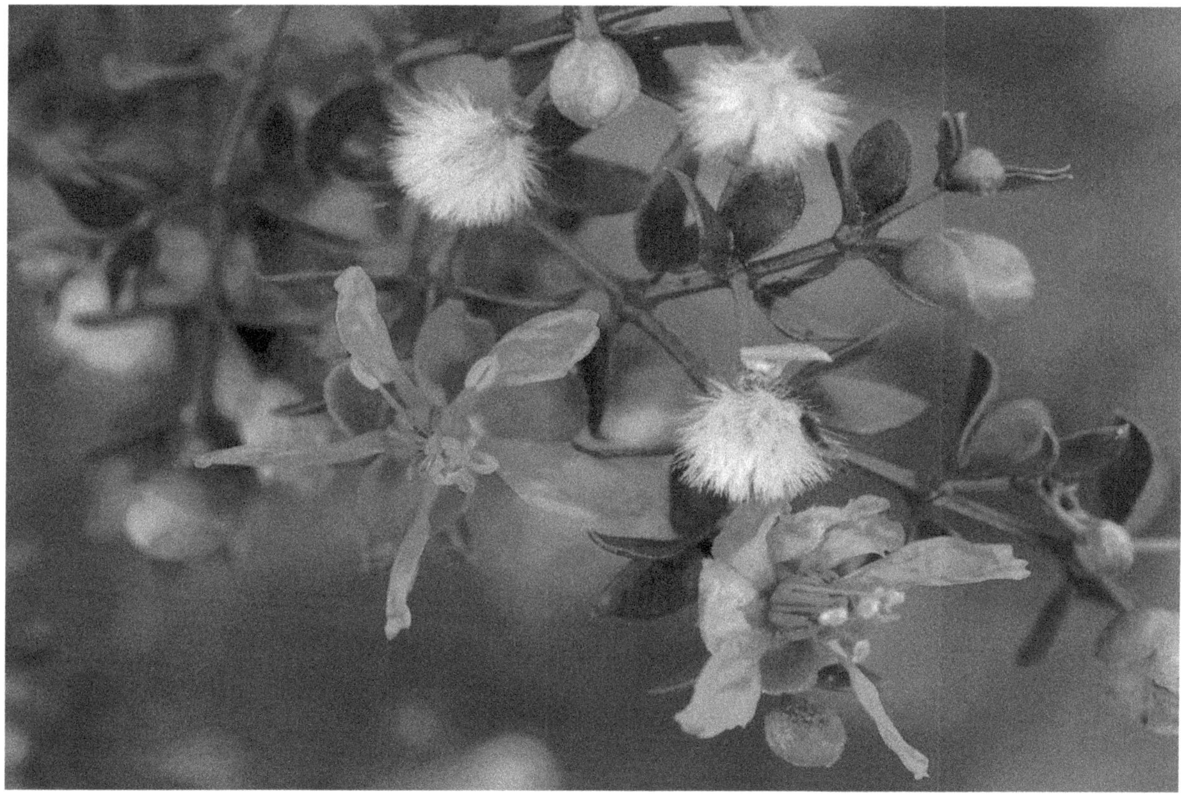

Chaparral (Larrea tridentate, goverrnadora) possesses a range of beneficial properties, including antimicrobial and antibacterial effects, as well as antitumor and anticancer properties. Additionally, it has been found to have antiulcerogenic and anti-inflammatory properties. In the past, chaparral has been utilized for its ability to eliminate parasites, combat sexually transmitted diseases, alleviate skin conditions such as eczema, psoriasis, rashes, and bruises, and act as an expectorant to relieve respiratory ailments like colds and bronchitis.

Origin: Mexico, Southwest North America

General commercial dose: One 500 mg capsule General dosage: One capsule two times daily

Cocolmeca

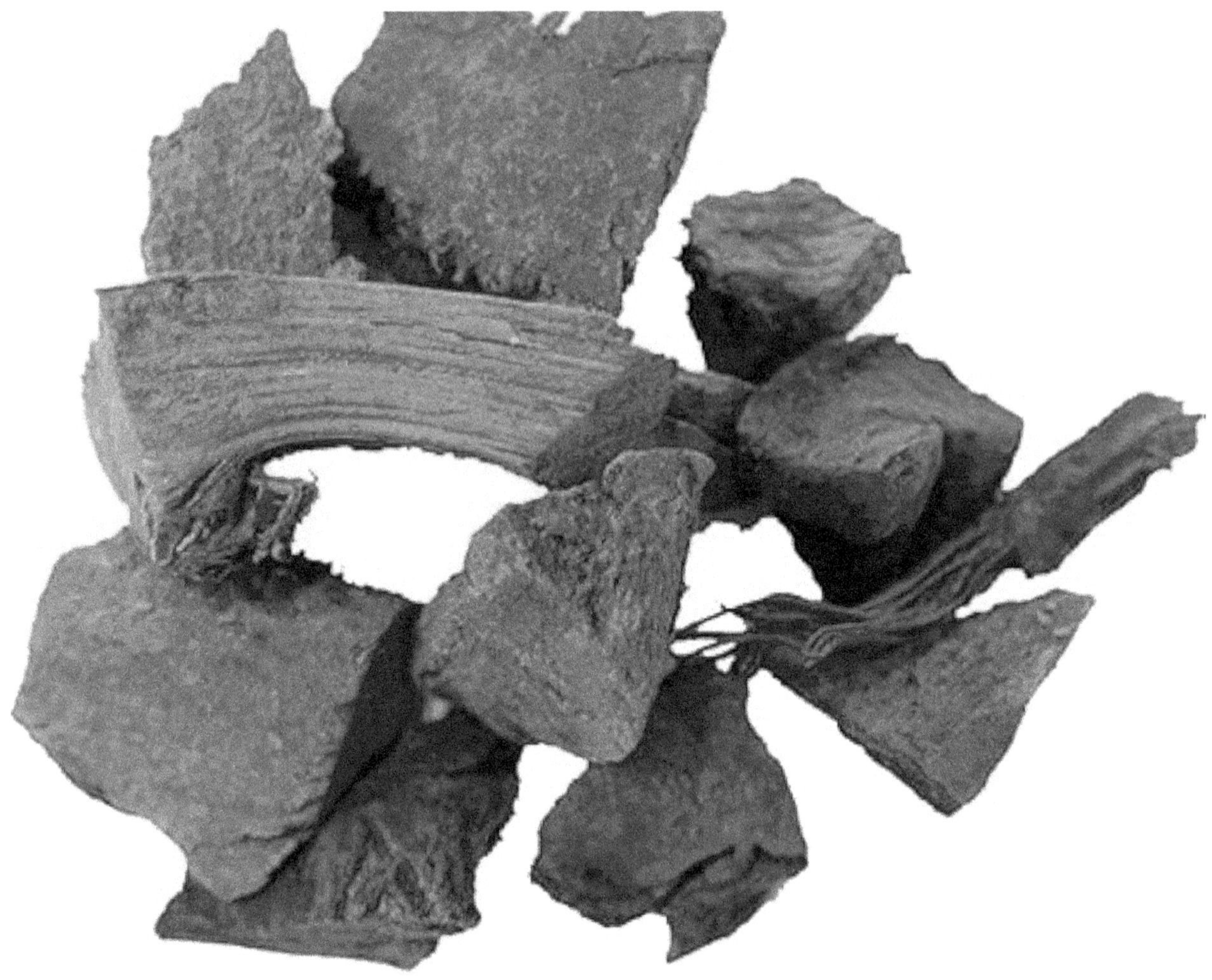

Cocolmeca (Smilax, Smilax regelii, Smilax aristolochiifolia, Jamaican sarsaparilla cocolmeca bark, cuculmeca) offers a variety of health benefits, such as reducing inflammation, preventing ulcers, fighting oxidative stress, combating cancer, promoting sweating, and aiding in urine production. Cocolmeca, a plant from the Smilax genus, has been scientifically proven to efficiently bind with toxins, aiding in their elimination from the bloodstream and the body. Cocolmeca has a long history of use in traditional medicine for treating a range of health issues, including skin conditions like psoriasis and leprosy, rheumatoid arthritis and joint pain, headaches, colds, and sexual impotence.

Origin: Mexico, Jamaica General commercial dose: One 450 mg capsule

General dosage: One capsule two times daily

Contribo

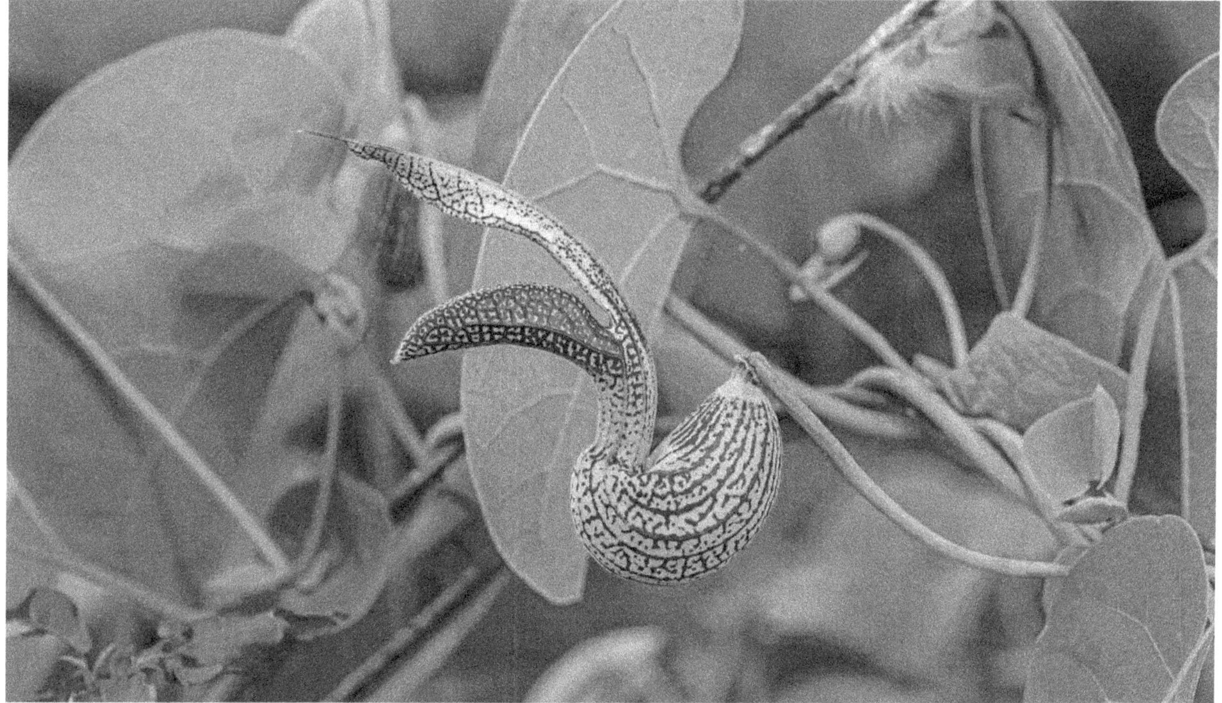

Contribo (Aristolochia, Aristolochia grandiflora, birthwort, duckflower, alcatraz, hierba del Indio) has been widely recognized for its extensive traditional medicinal use throughout history. It has been used to address arthritis and edema, enhance the immune system and white-blood-cell production, eliminate parasites, and treat snakebites.

Origin: South America

General commercial dose: Not used in commercial products (found to be poisonous)

(**Important medical note**: Contribo should be avoided by women who are pregnant or nursing. Contribo is known to have potential adverse effects on kidney function and should only be used under the guidance of a qualified and informed professional.

Damiana

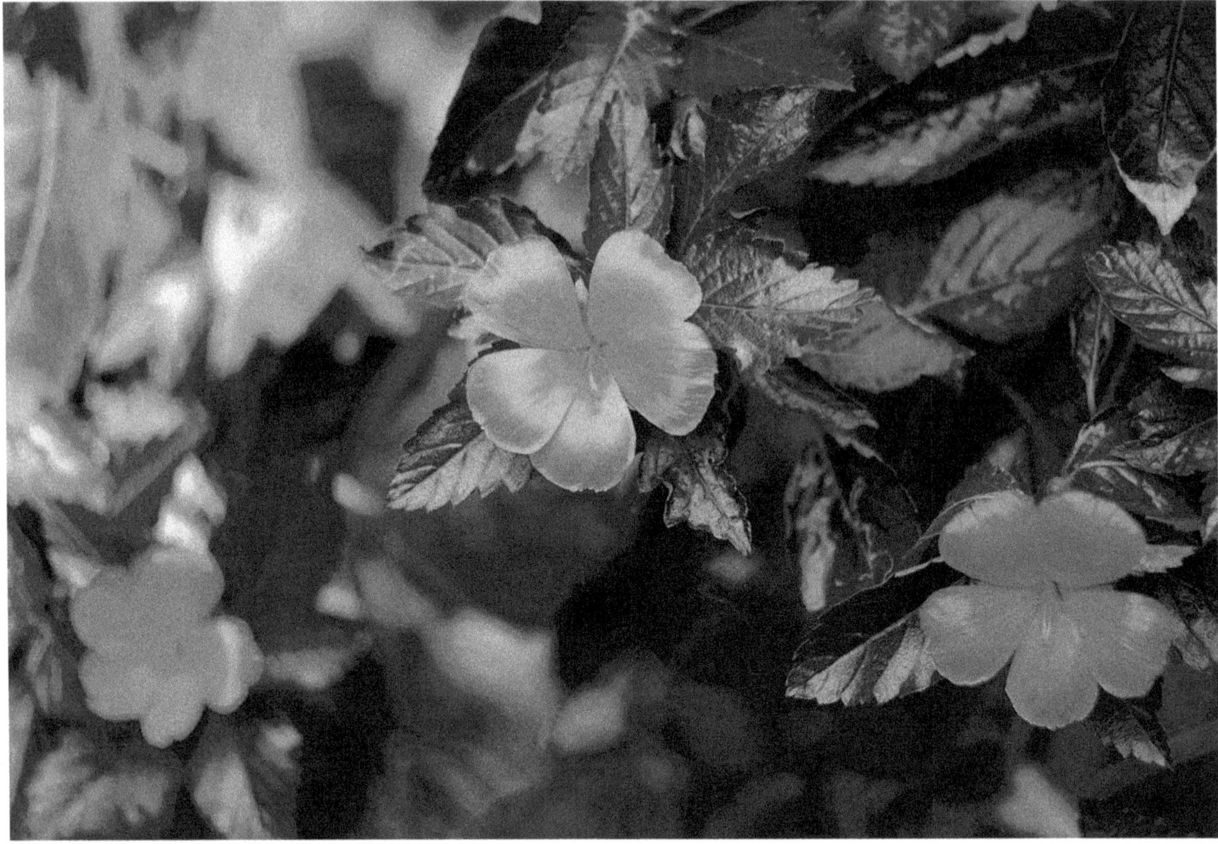

Damiana (Turnera diffusa, turnera, turnea aprodisiaca, damiana aphrodisiaca, damiana herb, damiana leaf) possesses properties that can help reduce anxiety and inhibit aromatase. Many individuals rely on damiana to enhance their sexual organs and increase their sexual drive and potency. The anti-aromatase property inhibits the conversion of androstenedione and estrone into estrogen. Damiana is commonly used to assist in managing estrogen-related conditions in women, such as breast cancer and fibroids. Women also find it helpful in managing hot flashes that occur during menopause. It additionally aids in maintaining hormonal balance, including supporting testosterone levels in men. Using Damiana can enhance oxygen delivery to the genitals, leading to a boost in libido. Damiana is also utilized for addressing depression, nervousness, and alleviating anxiety related to sexual dysfunction. Damiana has a stimulating effect on the intestinal tract, making it a valuable treatment for constipation.

Origin: Mexico, Central and South America, the Caribbean General commercial dose: One 400 mg capsule
General dosage: Two capsules two or three times daily

Elderberry

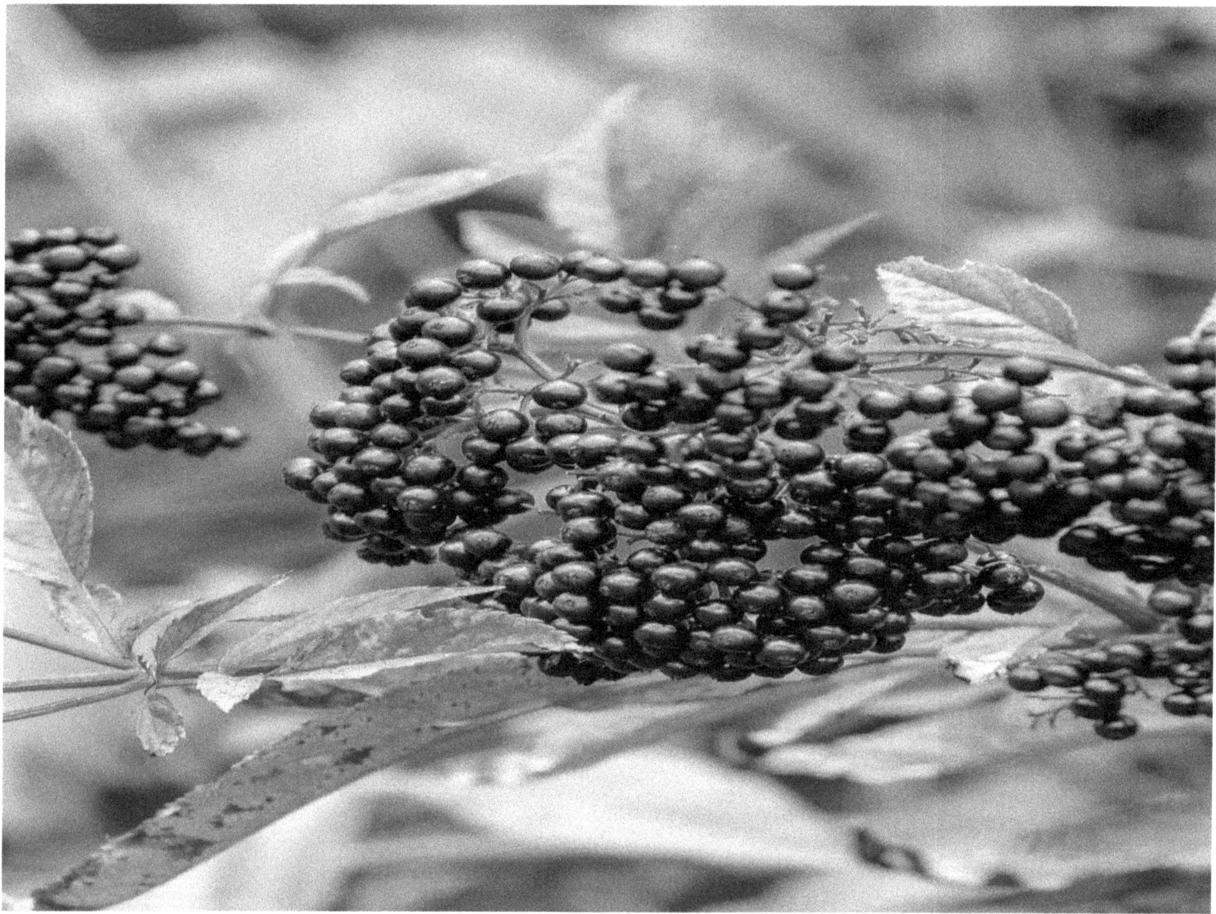

Elderberry, specifically the Sambucus variety, possesses remarkable properties that include anti-inflammatory, antiviral, anti-influenza, and anticancer effects. This product is commonly used to alleviate symptoms associated with colds, the flu, and allergies, as well as to help clear mucus from the respiratory system. Sambucus nigra is commonly used for its medicinal properties due to its non-toxic nature, unlike certain other species. Studies have demonstrated that Sambucus nigra has the ability to bind with the HINI virus, preventing its entry into cells.

Origin: America, Africa, Asia, Europe

General commercial dose: One 500 mg capsule General dosage: Two capsules two or three times daily

Eyebright

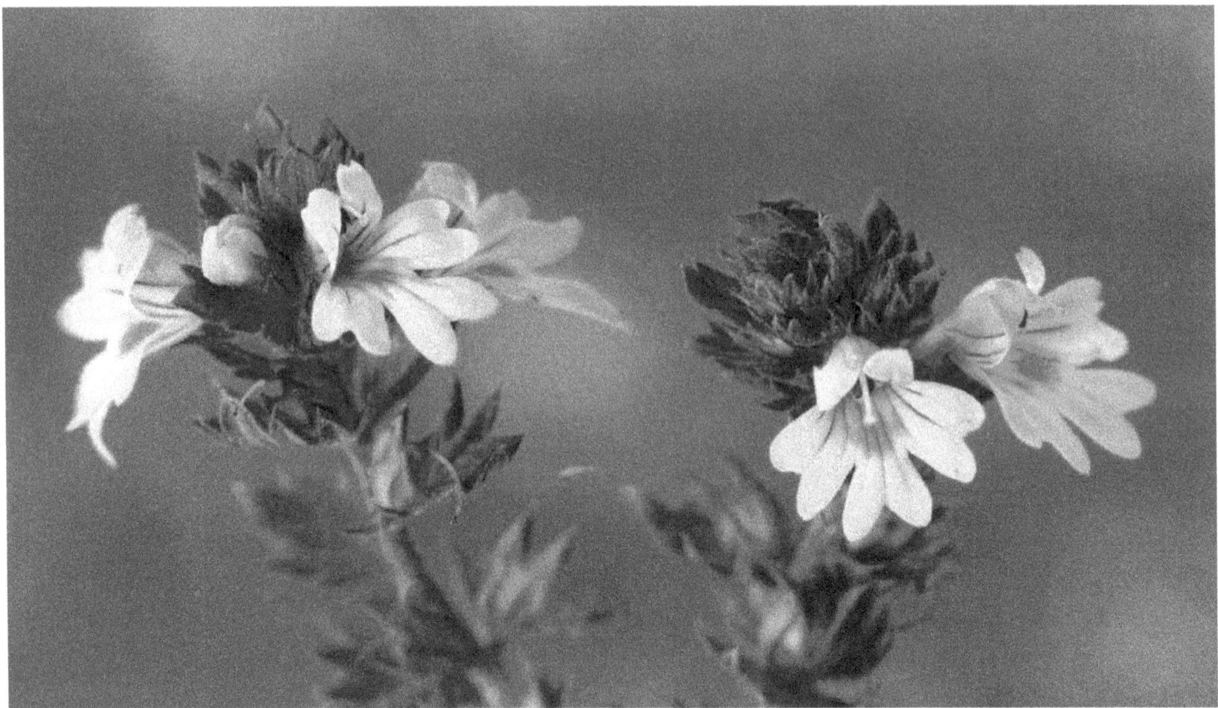

Eyebright, specifically Euphrasia officinalis and Euphrasia rostkoviana, possesses properties that can reduce inflammation and act as an antiseptic. It is commonly utilized as an eyewash to provide relief to the eye's mucous membrane and address long-lasting eye inflammation. Eyebright is commonly used as an antimicrobial to effectively treat bacterial infections such as conjunctivitis and blepharitis that affect the eye. Eyebright is commonly used as an astringent for treating wounds and reducing skin inflammation. Additionally, it is utilized internally to alleviate inflammation and address upper respiratory infections such as sinusitis and hay fever.

Origin: ~

Recommended dosage for commercial use: One capsule containing 450 mg Recommended dosage: Take two capsules once daily Basic mode: Infuse ½ teaspoon of eyebright herb in 8 oz. of boiled water for 15 minutes. Filter the mixture through cheesecloth into a container to separate any herb particles. Consider utilizing an eyewash cup for cleansing the eyes.

Position the eyewash cup over the eye you wish to cleanse. Adjust the angle of your head slightly to ensure that the wash fully covers your eye. For 20 seconds, gently move your eyes in different directions. Once you have finished cleaning one eye, simply dispose of the eyewash, replenish the eyewash cup, and proceed to clean the other eye.

Make sure to wash twice a day.

Guaco

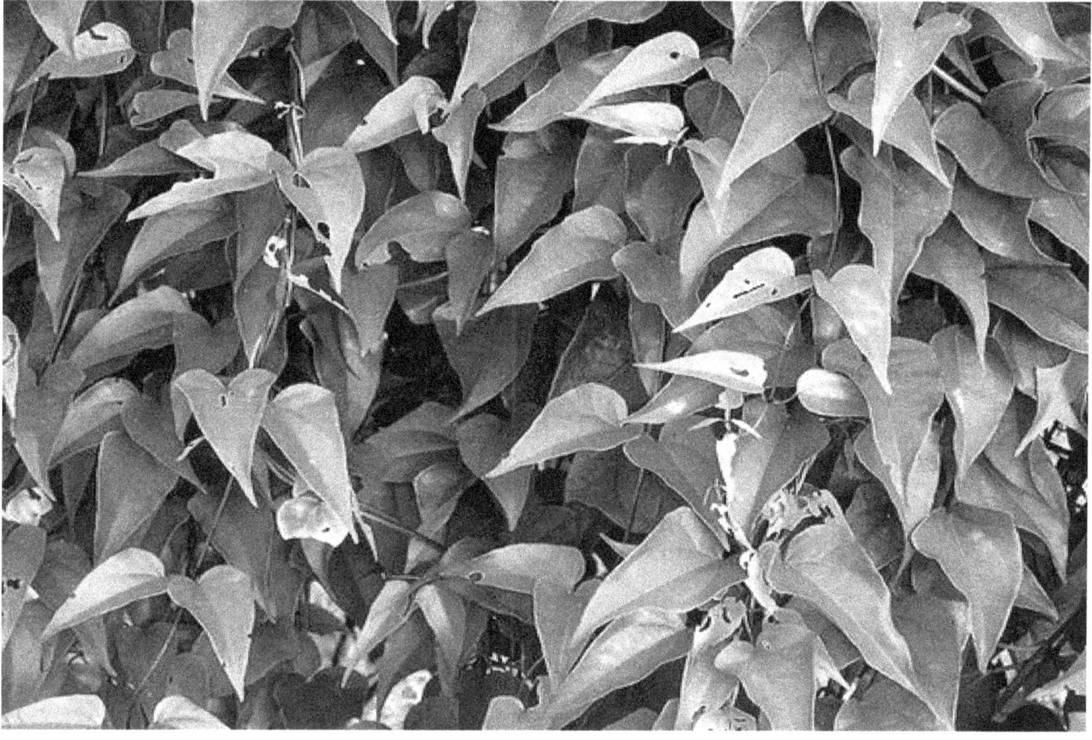

Guaco, also known as Mikania guaco, Mikania glomerata, guace, bejuco de finca, cepu, liane francois, matafinca, vedolin, cipó caatinga, huaco, or erva das serpentes, possesses properties that are anti-inflammatory, antiallergic, and bronchodilator in nature.

Guaco is commonly utilized in traditional medicine to address upper respiratory issues such as asthma, bronchitis, colds, and flu. It is commonly utilized to reduce inflammation associated with rheumatoid arthritis and digestive tract issues, as well as to combat Candida and yeast infections. Guaco has a content of approximately 10 percent coumarin, known for its blood-thinning properties.

Origin: Originating from South America and Jamaica Typical dosage: Guaco is commonly enjoyed as a tea, with a standard infusion of 4 oz. Regular infusion: Add 1 tablespoon of herb to 1 cup/8 oz. of boiling water. Allow the herb to infuse in the boiling water for 15–20 minutes.

Recommended dosage: 4 oz. two or three times daily Standard commercial dosage:

A single capsule containing 300 mg Recommended dosage: Take one capsule two or three times daily.

Huereque

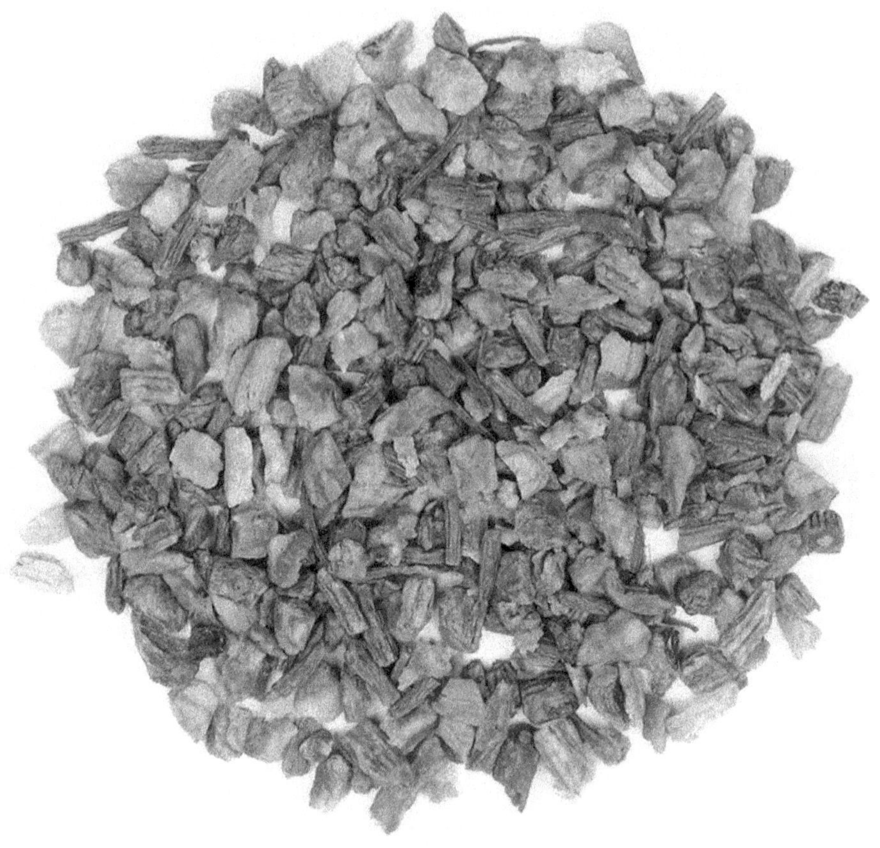

Huereque (Ibervillea sonorae, guareque, wareki, choyalhuani, wereke, big root, coyote melon, cowpie plant) possesses properties that have been found to be hypoglycemic, antiobesity, and antimicrobial in nature. Huereque is commonly utilized in traditional medicine for its potential benefits in managing blood-sugar levels, addressing diabetes, and aiding in weight reduction. It is utilized for nourishing and cleansing the pancreas.

Origin: Northwest Mexico

General commercial dose: One 500 mg capsule General dosage: One capsule three times daily with meals

Hombre Grande

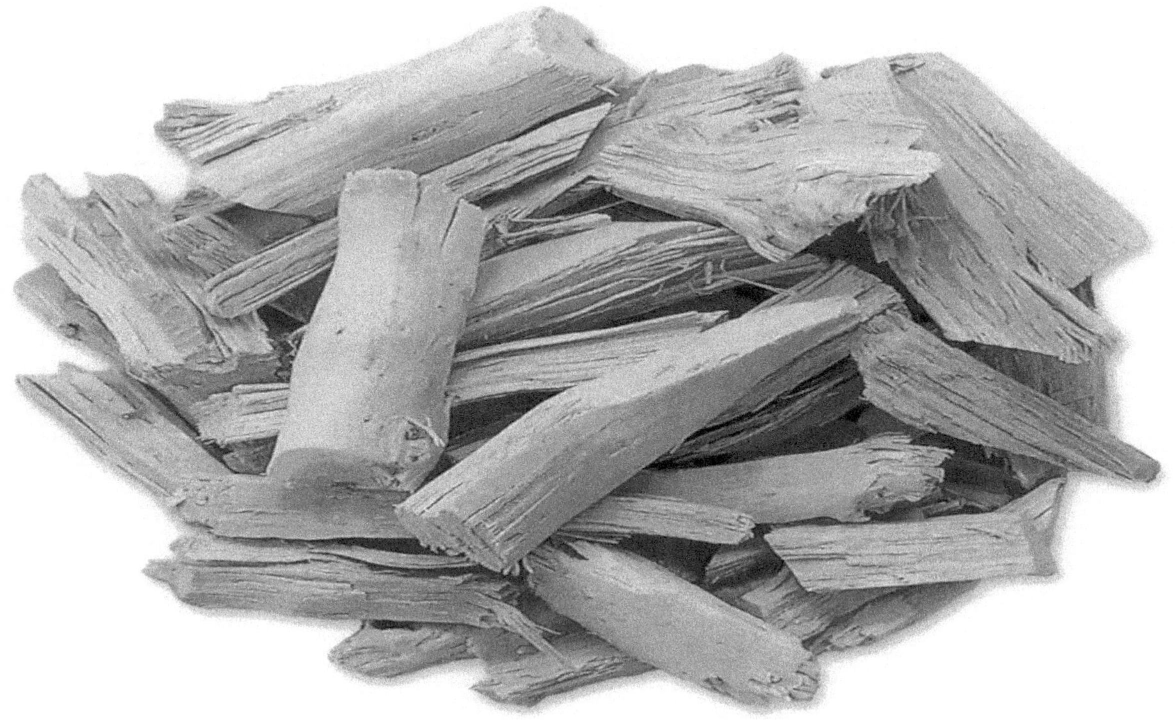

This powerful plant, known for its various names, has remarkable properties that can effectively combat fungi, ulcers, malaria, cancer, and insects.

Traditionally, Hombre grande has been utilized in medicine for topical treatment of measles and to address digestive issues like constipation, diarrhea, and intestinal parasite infections. Additionally, it has been utilized to aid in lowering body temperature. It is used to improve the functioning of the digestive tract, increase appetite, cleanse the blood, and stimulate enzyme production. Our product helps to restore the balance of flora in the digestive tract, which in turn supports a healthy immune system.

Origin: Originating from the Caribbean, Jamaica, Central and South America

Standard dosage: Take one capsule containing 450 mg Recommended dosage: Take one capsule three times a day. Traditionally, this herb was prepared as a tincture using the plant's bark. Grinders are now utilized to create a fine powder that can be consumed either in capsule form or by dissolving it in hot water.

Hops

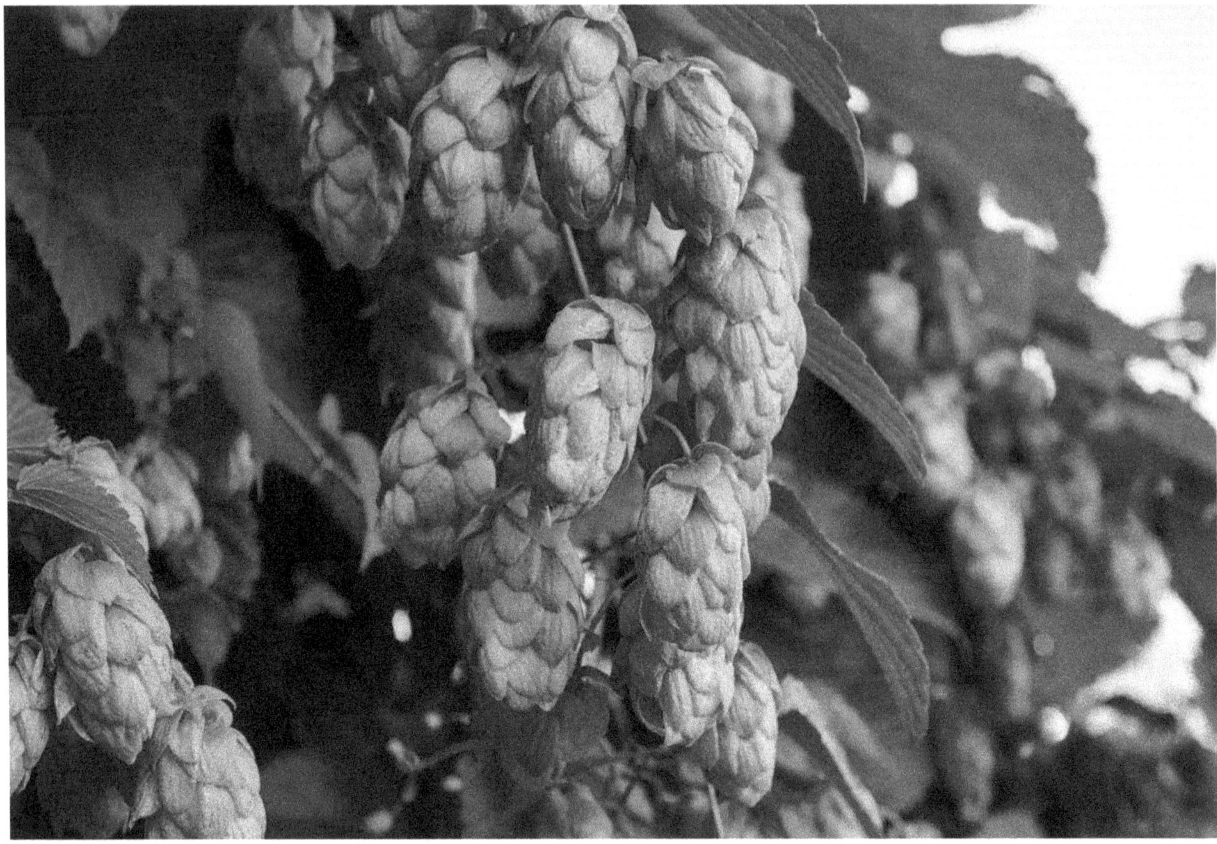

Hops (Humulus lupulus, lupulo) possesses antibacterial, anti-inflammatory, and anticancer properties. Hops has been utilized in traditional medicine for its various benefits. It is known to have anti-inflammatory properties, providing relief from pain and promoting digestion, urination, and appetite. Additionally, it has been used to treat rheumatic pains, infections, insomnia, and sleeping disorders. Hops is also believed to help reduce anxiety, tension, attention deficit hyperactivity disorder (ADHD), irritability, and nervousness.

Origin: Germany General commercial dose: One 310 mg capsule

General dosage: Two capsules once daily or one capsule twice daily

Hydrangea

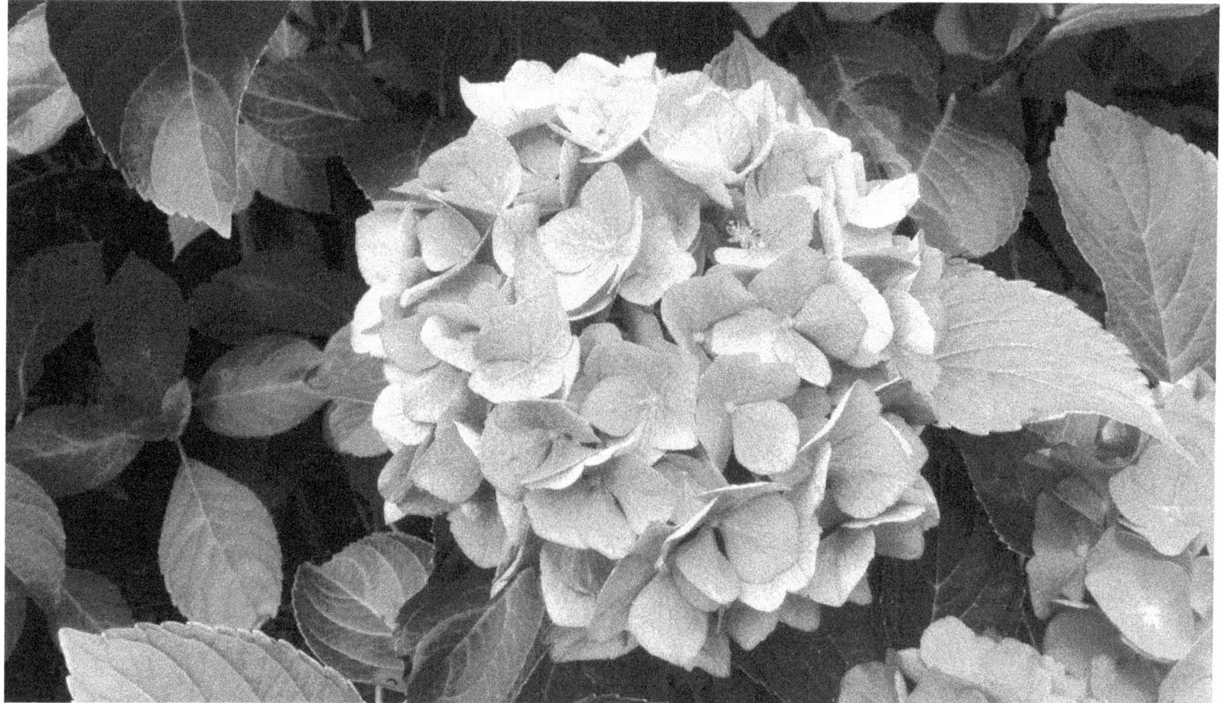

Hydrangea Root possesses a range of beneficial properties, including anti-inflammatory, lithotrophic, antiseptic, antiparasitic, and autoimmune effects. Hydrangea is valued for its hydrangin compound, renowned for its ability to dissolve calcium deposits in soft tissue. It has been traditionally used for the treatment of bladder and kidney disease, as well as for dissolving kidney stones and cleansing the lymphatic system. Chang Shan is commonly utilized in Chinese medicine due to its febriugine compound, which is known for its effectiveness in treating autoimmune diseases.

Origin: Northeastern Asia, Southwestern United States General commercial dose: One 400 mg capsule
General dosage: Two capsules two times daily

Lavender

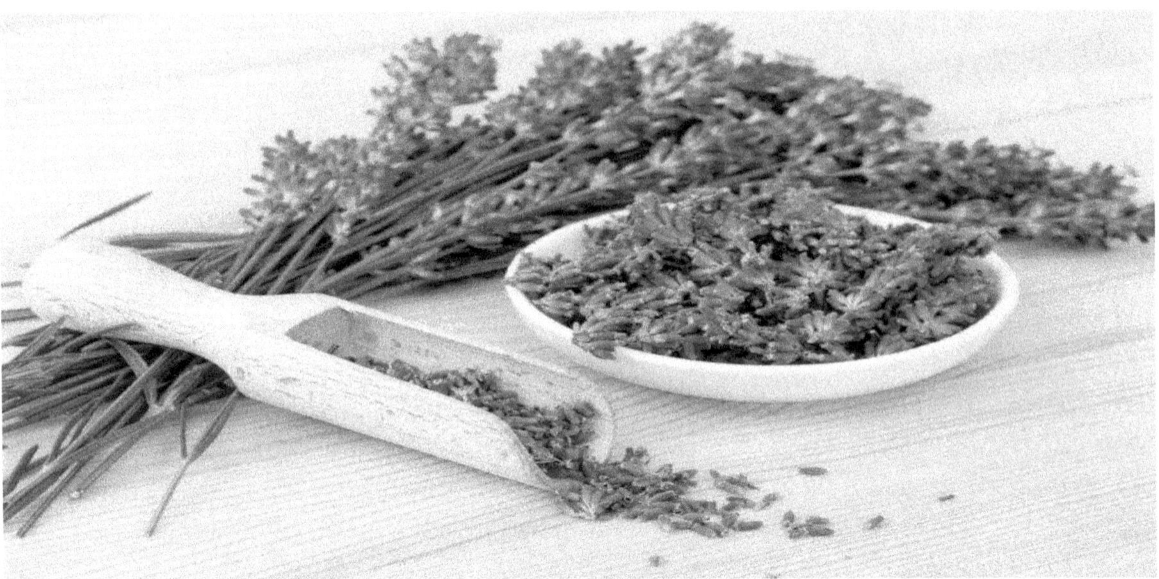

Lavender (Lavandula) offers a diverse array of advantageous properties, encompassing antifungal, antibacterial, analgesic, anti-inflammatory, anti-insomnia, anticonvulsant, antispasmodic, and antianxiety and antidepressant effects. Lavender is often used in traditional medicine to help with symptoms like restlessness, insomnia, nervousness, and depression. Lavender is often used to help relieve migraines, nerve pain, and joint pain. It is highly effective in relieving abdominal swelling caused by gas, upset stomach, nausea, loss of appetite, and vomiting.

Origin: Originating from various regions such as Africa, the Canary Islands, the Mediterranean, Asia, and India. Lavender is commonly used as an essential oil and is created through distillation. You will be left with pure lavender oil, but approximately 150 parts of lavender are required to produce 1 part of oil. (To produce 1 oz. of oil, approximately 150 oz. of lavender would be required.) The distilled lavender is mainly used for inhalation.

For a truly exquisite infusion of lavender, take some crushed fresh dried lavender and place it in a jar. Then, pour in just enough oil to completely cover the lavender. Coconut oil would enhance its medicinal properties. Make sure to leave some space in the jar to allow for proper air circulation. Place the jar in a spot that receives ample sunlight. One can expect to detect the scent of lavender in the oil after a period of forty-eight hours, although it is customary to allow the oil to bask in the sun for a duration of up to six weeks.

The lavender infusion can be utilized as a fragrant cologne or perfume, or as a soothing oil for relieving soreness and arthritis. Lavender is also enjoyed when ground up.

Standard commercial dosage: A single capsule containing 500 mg Recommended dosage: Take one capsule once to three times daily

Lily of the Valley

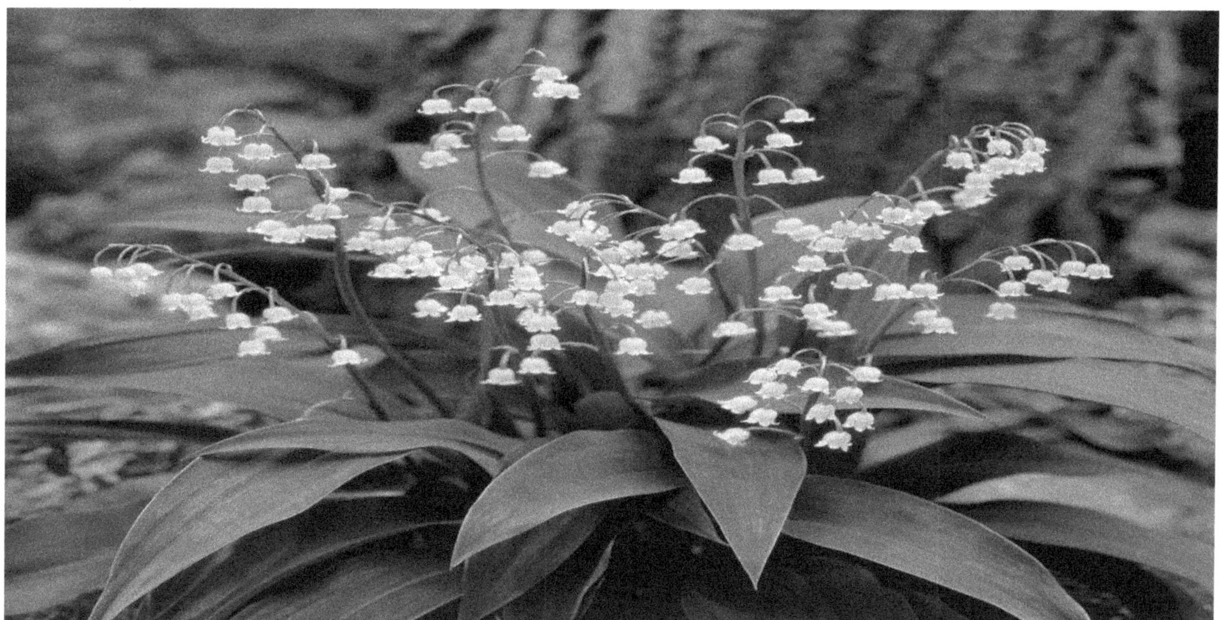

Lily of the valley, also known as Convallaria majalis, is a beautiful flower with various medicinal properties. It has been found to possess antiangiogenic, antitumor, and diuretic properties. Lily of the valley has a long history in traditional medicine, where it has been valued for its ability to support heart health and address conditions like heart failure and irregular heartbeat. The action of Lily of the valley is comparable to that of Digitalis, although it is derived from natural sources and is less concentrated, resulting in a milder effect. It is commonly prescribed for heart debility and dropsy. This mode enhances the delivery of oxygen to the heart, lowers blood pressure, and supports a weakened heart to beat at a more optimal pace, thereby improving its efficiency and strength.

Origin: Originating from Europe and Northern Asia

Standard dosage: Consume one tablespoon of the infusion daily. It may be challenging to find a commercially available bottled product, as lily of the valley is typically administered by a trained herbalist or medical professional.

A delightful infusion can be created by adding ½ oz. of lily of the valley to one pint of boiling water. The infusion is left to steep until it cools down. It is best to store it in an airtight glass container in a cool, dark place. It is recommended to avoid straining the herb and instead, gently shake the mixture before using a tablespoon of it.

Nettle

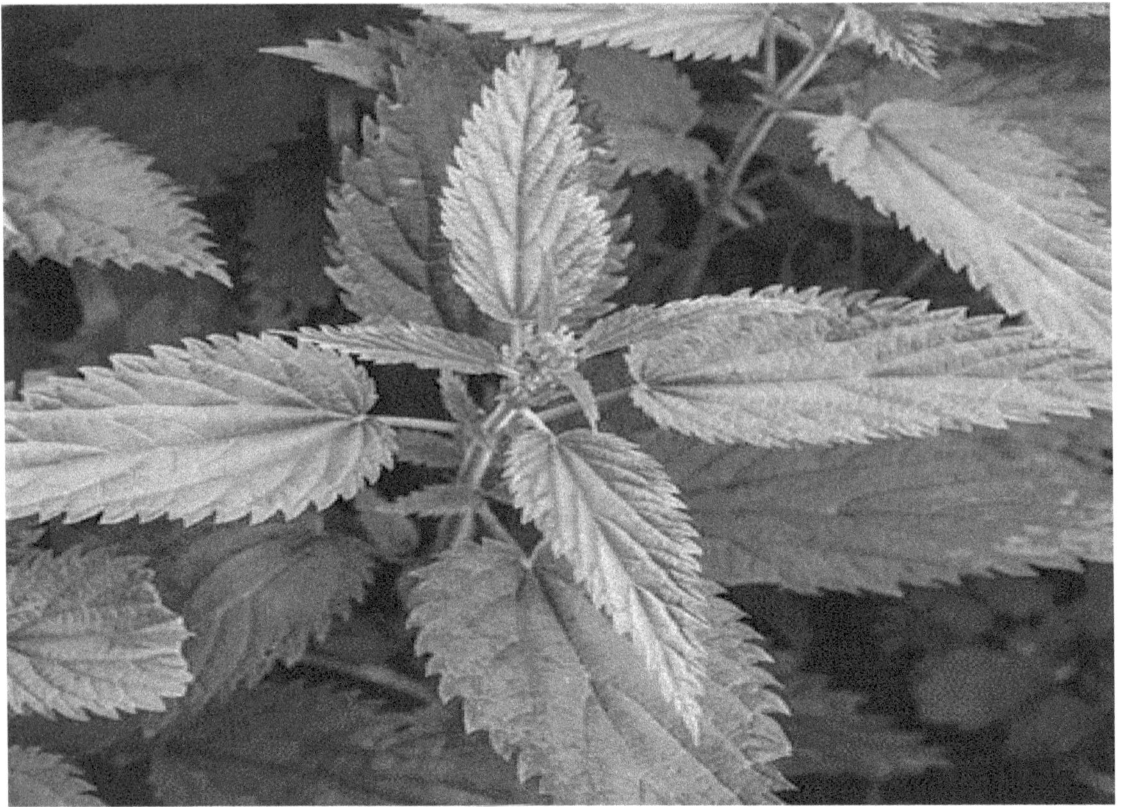

Nettle (Urtica dioica, ortiga, stinging nettle) possesses a range of beneficial properties, including anti-inflammatory, anticancer, diuretic, antioxidant, antimicrobial, antiulcer, and analgesic activities.

Nettle root is commonly utilized to support prostate health, promote joint comfort, and act as a natural diuretic and astringent. Nettle leaves have various applications, including addressing arthritis, sore muscles, hair loss, anemia, poor circulation, diabetes, enlarged spleen, allergies, eczema and rash, and asthma. Nettle is commonly utilized to promote overall well-being and cleanse the bloodstream.

Origin: Native to North Africa, Asia, and Western North America Nettle Leaf

Standard dosage: Take one 435 mg capsule for commercial use or two capsules two times daily for general use. Contains Nettle Root. Standard commercial dosage: A single capsule containing 400 mg Recommended dosage: Take two capsules once or twice daily

Nopal

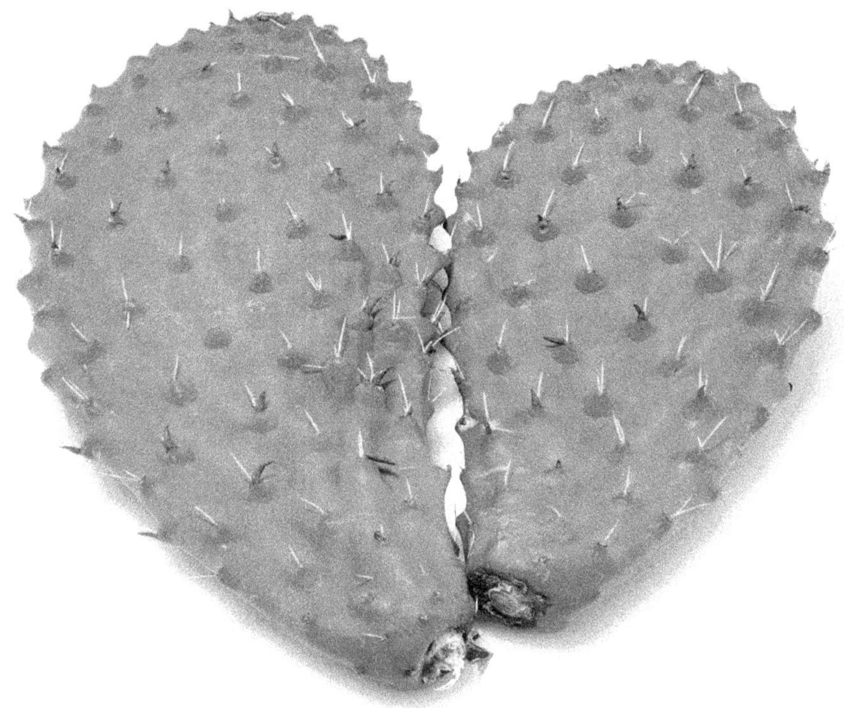

The paddle of the Opuntia cactus, also known as prickly pear or nopal cactus, is the site where the prickly-pear fruit is produced. Nopal contains a wide range of phytochemicals, antioxidants, vitamins, and minerals. It has proven to be highly effective in treating a range of conditions including type 2 diabetes, high cholesterol, obesity, alcohol hangover, colitis, diarrhea, and viral infections.

Origin: Mexico, Central America, the Caribbean, Western United States, Eastern United States

General commercial dose: One 400 mg capsule General dosage: Two capsules two times daily

Prodigiosa

Prodigiosa (Brickellia canvanillesi, prodigiosa, amula, hamula, calea zacatechichi, dream herb, cheech, bitter grass) has been traditionally used in medicine to promote the stimulation of pancreas and liver secretions. It is believed to enhance bile synthesis and facilitate the evacuation of bile from the gallbladder. Prodigiosa is an effective remedy for a range of ailments, including diarrhea, stomach pain, gallbladder disease, and diabetes. It helps to regulate blood-sugar levels, providing relief and promoting overall well-being. Prodigiosa is an effective remedy for relieving headaches and reducing fever. Prodigiosa possesses remarkable qualities that can help alleviate anxiety and promote vivid dreaming.

Origin: Southwestern North America, specifically New Mexico Typical dosage: Prodigiosa is commonly enjoyed as an infusion or tea, with a recommended serving size of 2-4 ounces for a standard infusion.

Regular infusion: Use 1 tablespoon of herb for every 1 cup/8 oz. of boiling water. Allow the herb to infuse in the boiling water for 15–20 minutes.

Recommended dosage: Take twice daily, once in the morning and once in the evening Recommended capsule dosage: Take one capsule containing 400 mg Recommended capsule dosage: Take one capsule twice daily (Begin with a lower dose if needed)

Red Clover

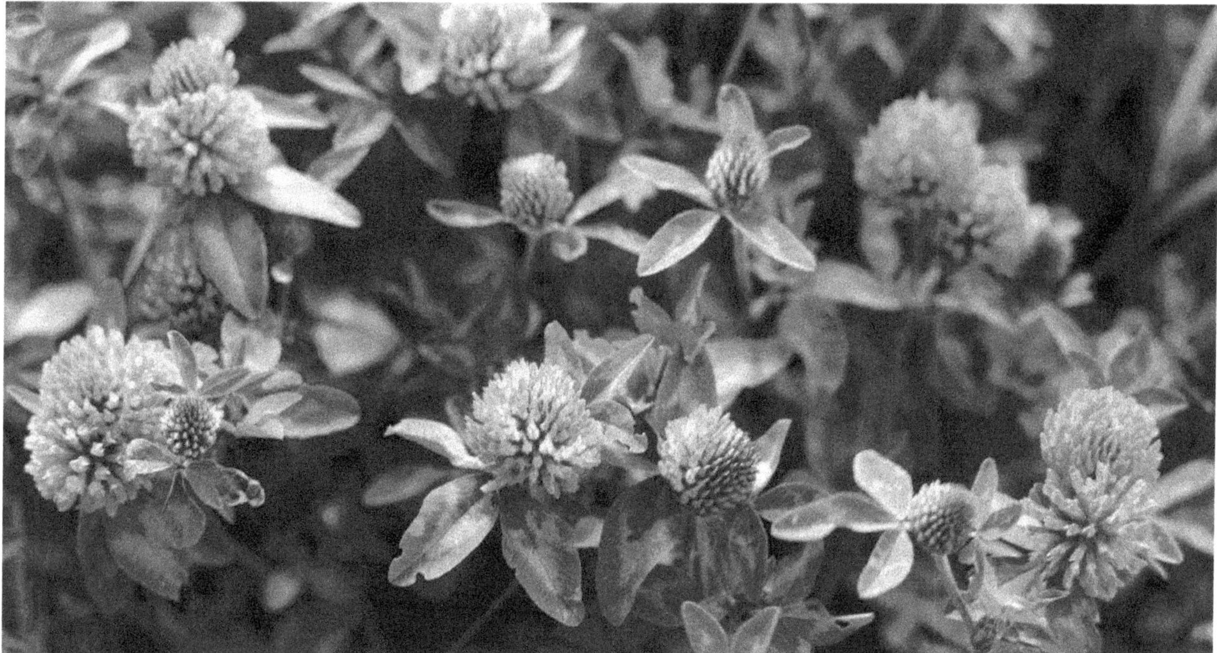

Red clover, scientifically named Trifolium pratense, is a versatile plant with numerous advantageous qualities. These effects encompass a range of benefits, such as fighting cancer, promoting urine production, aiding in cough relief, inducing relaxation, reducing inflammation, and preventing the buildup of plaque in arteries. Red clover is often used for its estrogenic properties, which can provide relief from symptoms related to menopause. Red clover possesses the remarkable capability of cleansing the blood and aiding in the removal of calcification from soft tissues. It also helps in purifying the lymphatic system by eliminating waste from lymph fluid.

Origin: Northwest Africa, Western Asia

General commercial dose: One 400 mg capsule General dosage: Two capsules once daily or one capsule twice daily

Rhubarb Root

Rhubarb root (Rheum palmatum, Chinese rhubarb, Turkish rhubarb, Indian rhubarb, Russian rhubarb, R. tanguticum and R. officinale - da-huang) has antioxidant, heavy-metal chelation, anticancer, and antibacterial properties. Rhubarb root is used regulate the digestive tract to treat digestive issues that include diarrhea, constipation, stomach pain, and acid reflux. Rhubarb root softens stool to ease bowel movements and reduces pain from hemorrhoids and tears of the lining of the anus. Rhubarb root is used to treat kidney stones and kidney disease, to chelate heavy metals, to remove acids and mucus, and to intracellularly cleanse cells.

Origin: China General commercial dose: One 500 mg capsule General dosage: One capsule two or three times daily.

Sage

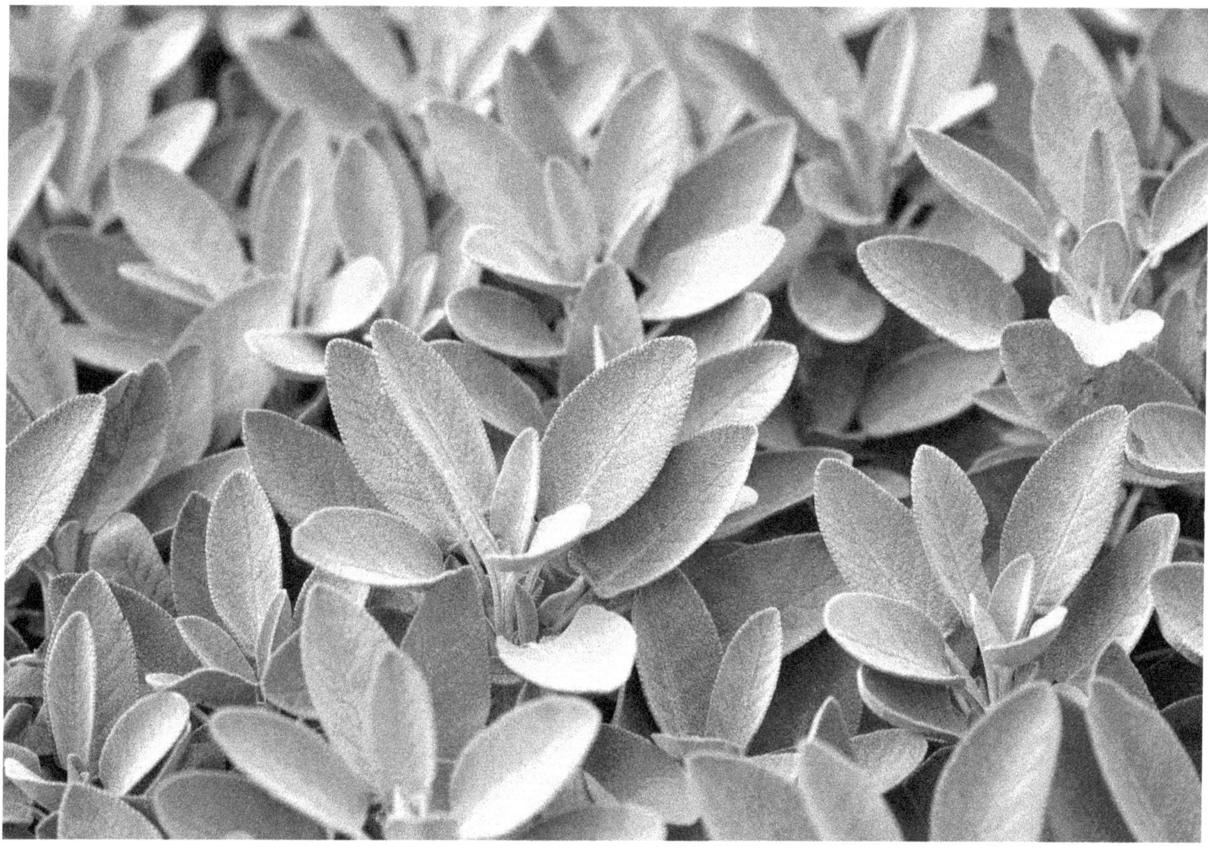

Sage (Salvia officinalis) offers a multitude of health benefits, such as its ability to provide antioxidant support, fight against harmful microorganisms, reduce inflammation, combat tumors, alleviate diarrhea, and aid in weight management. Sage has been discovered to have a beneficial effect on cholesterol levels, enhancing the equilibrium between LDL and HDL cholesterol. Sage has a long history of being utilized in medicine for various purposes, including memory enhancement, relief from menopausal hot flashes, reduction of gastrointestinal inflammation, support for the pancreas, and management of diabetes.

Origin: Mediterranean General commercial dose: One 500 mg capsule

General dosage: Two capsules once daily or one capsule twice daily

Santa Maria

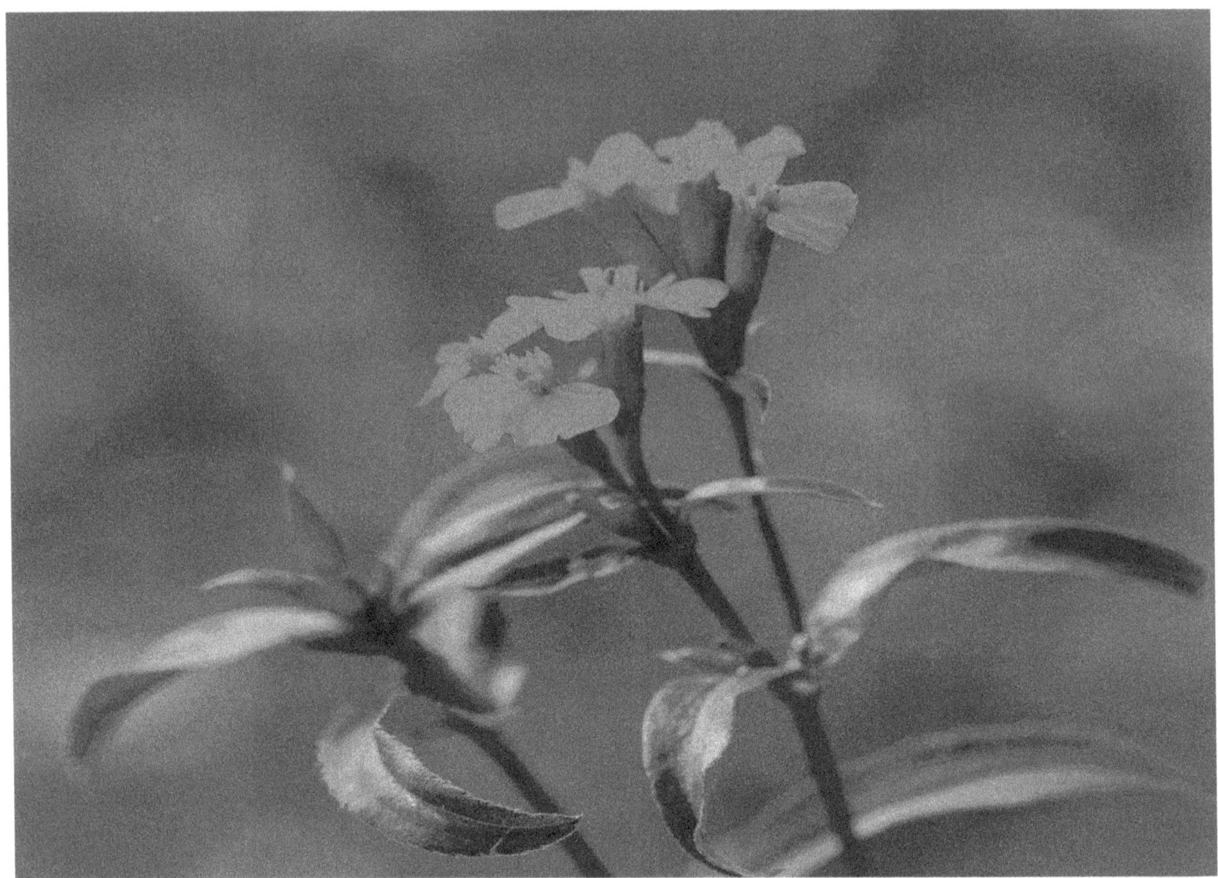

Santa Maria, also known as Tagetes lucida, pericón, hierbanis, yerbanís, Mexican marigold, or Mexican tarragon, offers a variety of advantageous properties. These include its ability to combat fungal and bacterial infections, its potential to alleviate depression, its antioxidant and pain-relieving qualities, and its anti-inflammatory benefits. Santa Maria is frequently used in traditional medicine to effectively treat various ailments, such as diarrhea, abdominal pains, respiratory infections, rheumatism, and inflammatory skin diseases. Santa Maria is renowned for its psychoactive properties and is frequently utilized to induce a sense of calmness and tranquility.

Origin: Central America, Mexico General dose: Santa Maria is usually consumed as an infusion/tea to enhance dreams and visualization—2–4 oz. standard infusion. Standard infusion: I tablespoon herb to I cup/8 oz. of boiling water. Steep the herb in the boiling water for I5–20 minutes.

General commercial dose: One 400 mg capsule General dosage: One or two capsules one or two times daily

Sapo

Sapo (Eryngium carlinae, yerba del sapo, hierba del sapo, grass frog, grass toad) has hypolipidemic, antioxidant, and anti-inflammatory properties. Sapo is used in traditional medicine to lower cholesterol and triglyceride levels in the blood and arteries. Sapo is used to treat gallstones and kidney stones.

Origin: Central America, Mexico General commercial dose: One 400 mg capsule General dosage: Two capsules two or three times daily with meals

Sarsaparilla

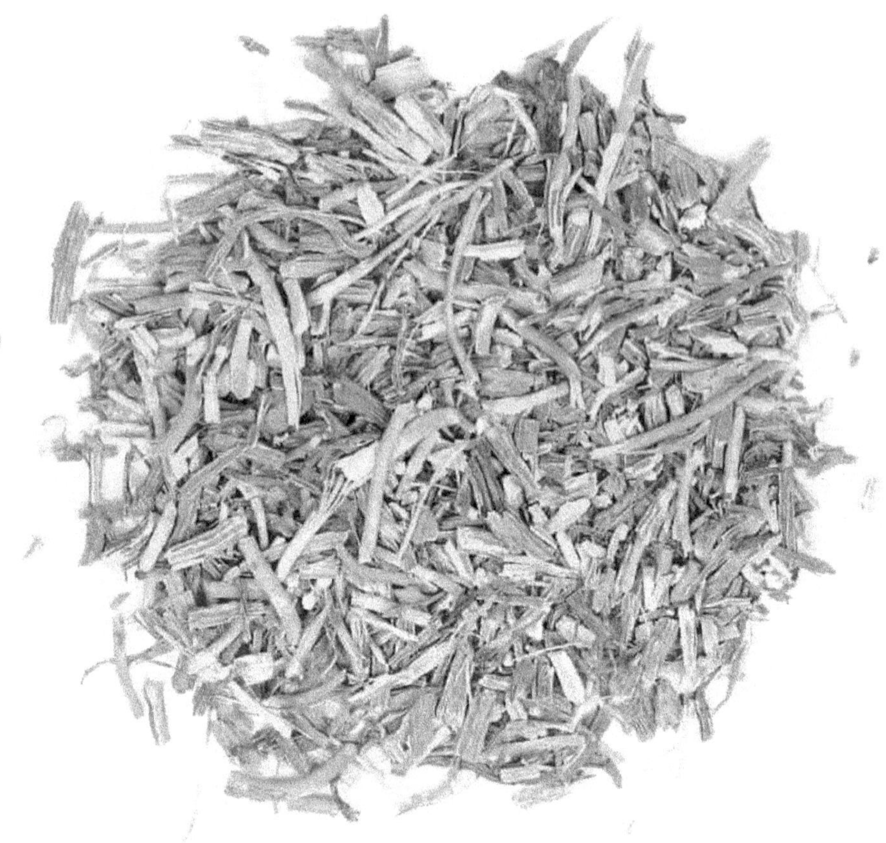

There are two species of plant, Smilax or Hemidesmus indicus that are commonly known as sarsaparilla. Smilax originates from South America, while Hemidesmus indicus hails from India. Interestingly, these two plants share several common properties. They possess a range of beneficial properties, including anti-inflammatory, antiulcer, antioxidant, anticancer, diaphoretic, and diuretic effects. Sarsaparilla has been proven to effectively bind with toxins, facilitating their elimination from the bloodstream and the body. Sarsaparilla has long been utilized in traditional medicine to address a range of health concerns, including skin conditions such as psoriasis and leprosy, rheumatoid arthritis and joint discomfort, headaches, colds, and issues related to sexual potency.

Origin: Mexico, Jamaica, India General commercial dose: One 450 mg capsule General dosage: One capsule two times daily

Sea Moss

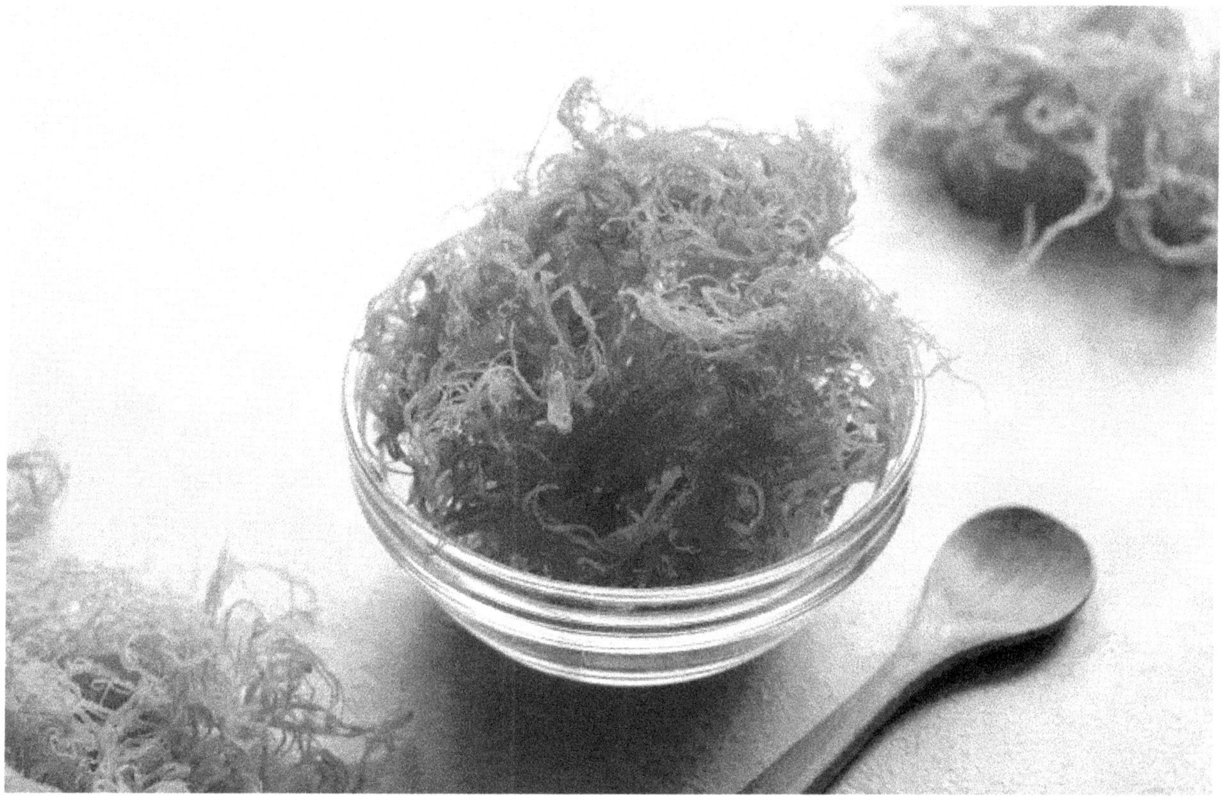

Sea moss (Chondrus crispus, Irish moss) possesses antibacterial, anti-inflammatory, and laxative properties. Sea moss is known for its soothing properties that can help alleviate irritation in mucous membranes caused by various conditions such as colds, coughs, bronchitis, tuberculosis, gastric ulcers, and intestinal problems. Sea moss is commonly utilized to promote joint and skin health, while its abundant array of nutrients acts as a natural mineral supplement.

Origin: Atlantic Ocean coastal area General commercial dose: One 400 mg (powder) capsule

General dosage: One capsule two times daily (Commercial doses vary greatly, because the properties of sea moss make it more of a natural nutritional supplement rather than a medicinal herb. Sea moss is used in greater quantities to make seamoss beverages and gels.)

Sensitiva

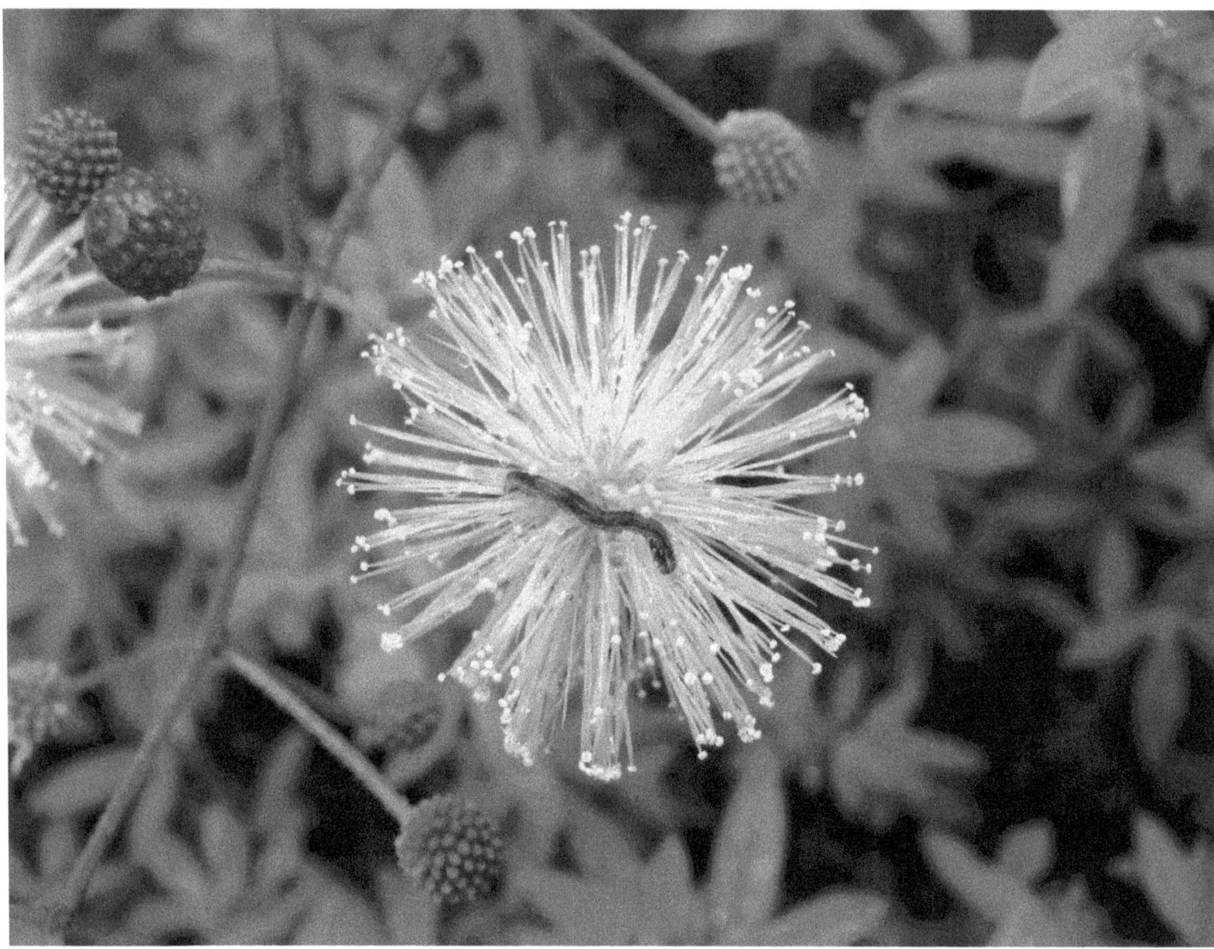

Sensitiva (Mimosa sensitiva, Mimosa pudica) possesses a wide range of beneficial properties, including antidepressant, anticonvulsant, antibacterial, diuretic, antioxidant, anti-inflammatory, and aphrodisiac effects. Sensitiva is commonly employed in traditional medicine to alleviate discomfort associated with hemorrhoids and arthritis, halt bleeding, and address uterine infections. Sensitiva is also known for its ability to enhance sexual desire and libido.

Origin: Central America General commercial dose: One 500 mg capsule

General dosage: One capsule two times daily

Shea Butter

Shea butter (Vitellaria paradoxa, Butyrospermum paradoxa, Butyrospermum parkii) is the nut is the shea tree Vitellaria paradoxa and is a traditional African plant food. It is popularly used for skin treatment. Shea butter made from the shea nut is rich in skin protective fatty acids, nutrients, and phytonutrients. It is used to moisturize the skin, increase elasticity, and treat conditions like blemishes, wrinkles, sunburn, eczema, and small wounds.

Origin: Africa Application: Shea butter is used as a cream and is applied directly to the skin.

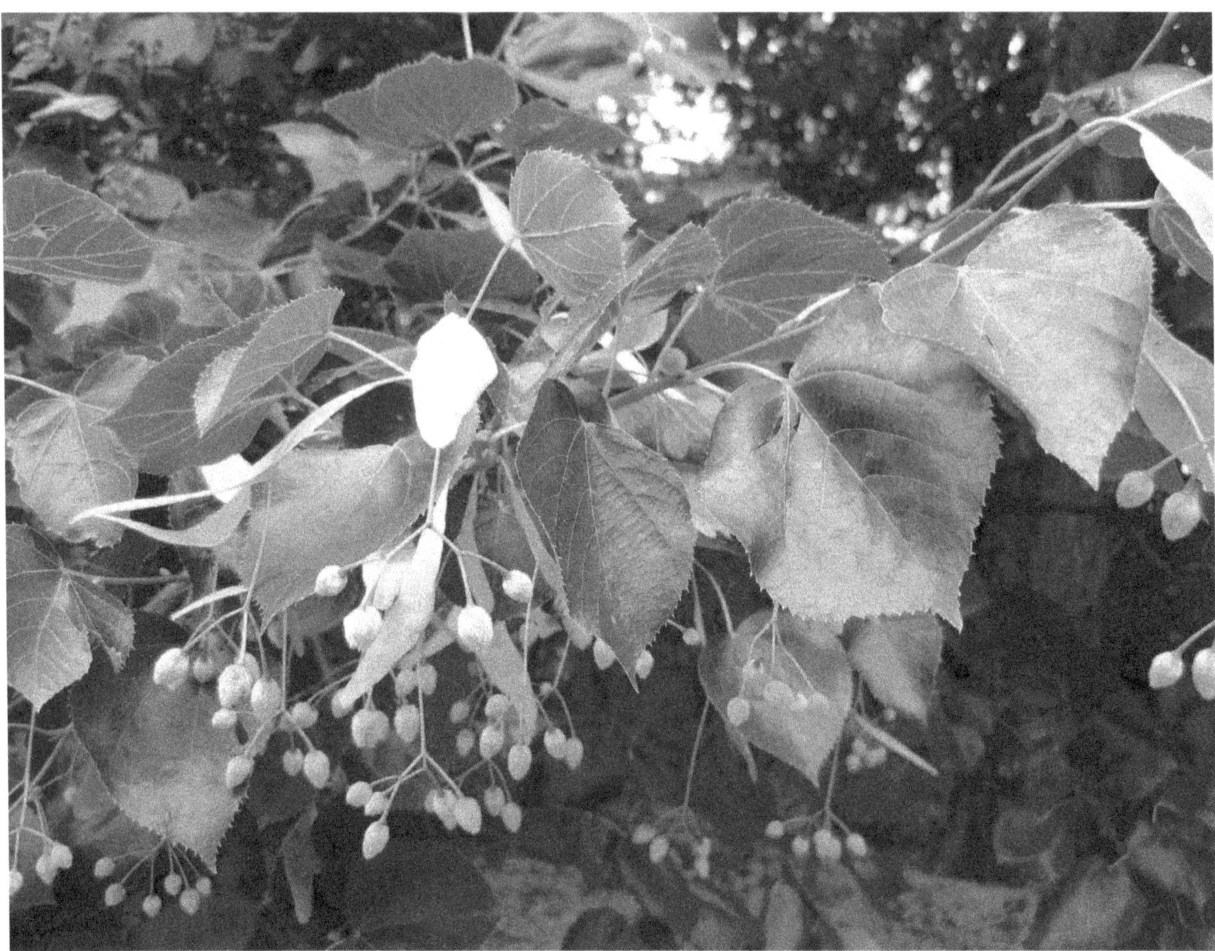

Tila (Tilia, linden, basswood) possesses a range of beneficial properties, including antioxidant, neuroprotective, anticonvulsant and antiseizure, antispasmodic, anti-inflammatory, anticancer, and diuretic properties. Linden has been utilized in traditional medicine for its potential benefits in supporting the immune system, promoting relaxation, alleviating depression, and addressing various conditions such as insomnia, fever, headaches, migraines, inflammatory skin conditions, and issues related to the liver and gallbladder.

Origin: North America, Asia, Europe

General commercial dose: One 500mg capsule General dosage: One capsule two or three times daily

Urtila Oil

Extracted from the nettle plant, Urtila oil is commonly used as a hair conditioner and to promote oil production in the scalp.

Valerian

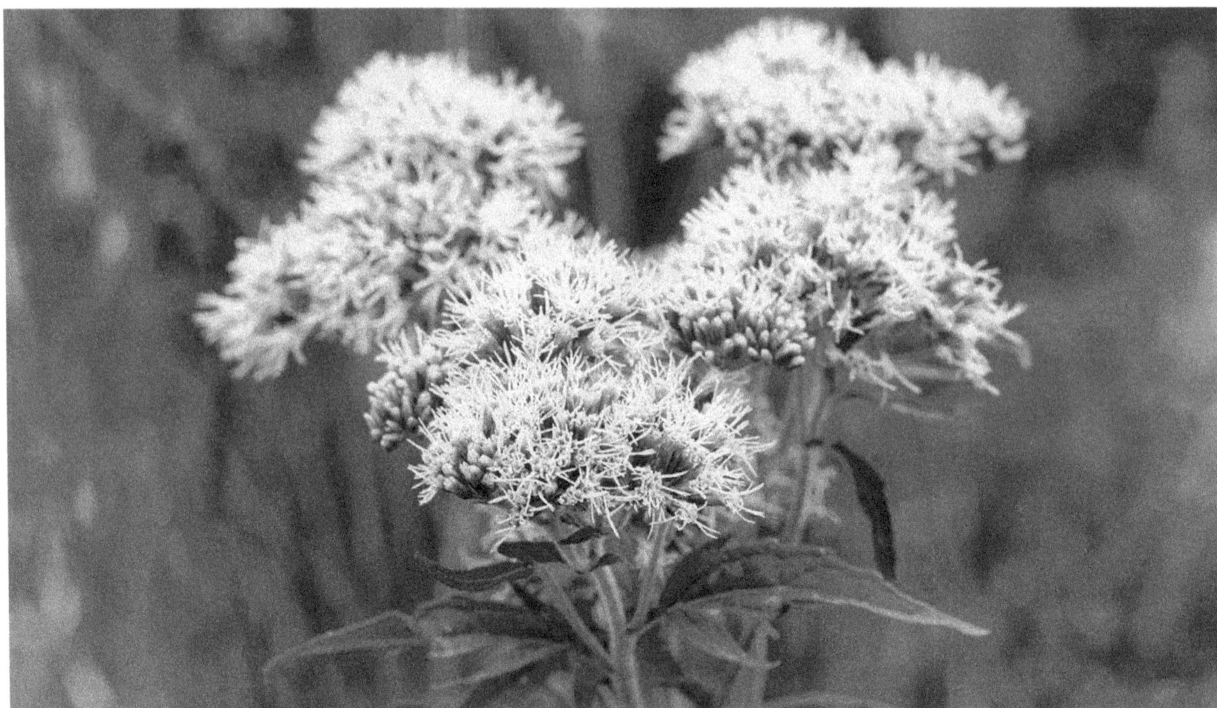

Valerian (Valerianu officinalis L Veleriana, valerian, capon's tail, all-heal, garden heliotrope, English valerian, Vermont valeria, setwall, wild valerian) possesses calming, anti-seizure, anxiety-reducing, and mood-enhancing properties. It provides relief from feelings of anxiety, nervousness, exhaustion, headaches, and hysteria.

Valerian is commonly used for its relaxing and uterine-strengthening properties.

Origin: Asia, Europe General commercial dose: One 500 mg capsule

General dosage: Two or three capsules before bedtime

Yellow Dock

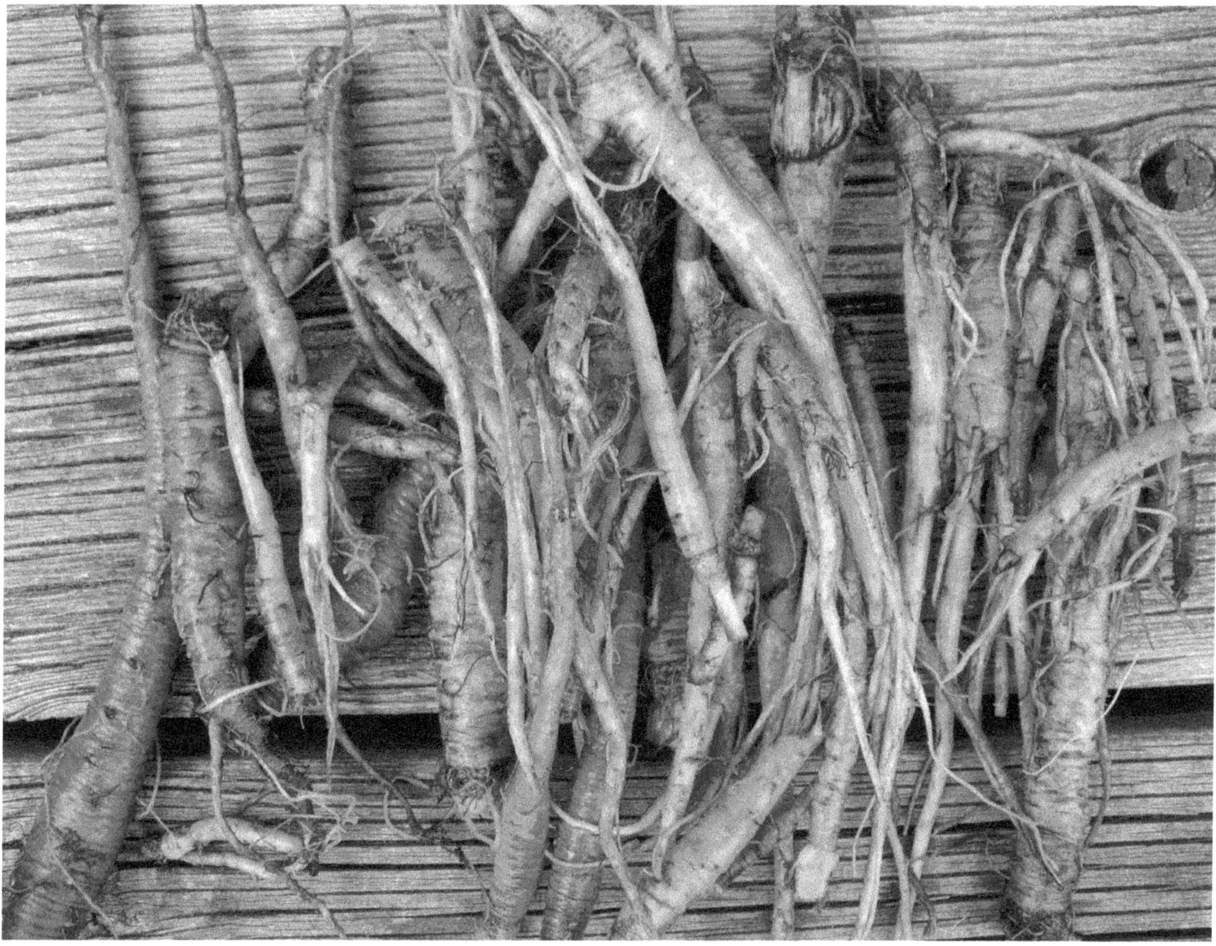

Yellow dock root, also known as Rumex crispus or curly dock, offers a multitude of health benefits. It has antioxidant, antimicrobial, antibacterial, anti-inflammatory, and analgesic and antipyretic effects. Yellow dock supports the production of bile, aiding in the digestion of fat and promoting regular bowel movements for a healthy digestive tract. Yellow dock has been used for centuries in traditional medicine for its believed ability to purify the blood, detoxify the liver and gallbladder, and support a well-functioning lymphatic system.

Origin: Africa, Western Asia, Europe General commercial dose: One 500mg capsule

General dosage: Two capsules two times daily (Medical caution: consult a physician if you have a history of kidney stones.

Yohimbe

Yohimbe (Corvanthe yohimbe, Pausinystalia johimbe, yohimbe bark, yohimbine) has antiobesity, antidepressant, and libidoenhancing properties. Yohimbe is used in traditional medicine to increase sexual desire and to reverse erectile impotence. Though yohimbe is used more often for male libido, it is also effective in increasing female sexual desire and performance.

Yohimbe is a ground herb derived from the bark. Yohimbine serves as the active component in Yohimbe, which manufacturers extract and sell as a concentrated extract. It is also artificially produced Yohimbine is not considered to be a natural option and is generally not recommended. The ground bark is not as strong as the extract, but it is a safer option to consider. Using larger doses of ground yohimbe bark is necessary to achieve the same level of effectiveness as yohimbine. However, the potency of the natural yohimbine alkaloid found in yohimbe is incredibly high, requiring only a small amount to enhance libido. When buying commercial capsules, it's important to check the ingredients and ensure they contain yohimbe bark instead of extract.

Origin: Western and Central Africa

General (bark) commercial dose:

One 500 mg (bark) capsule General (bark) dosage: One capsule two to three times daily with water. Its effect builds in the body over time. You may want to start with one capsule daily.

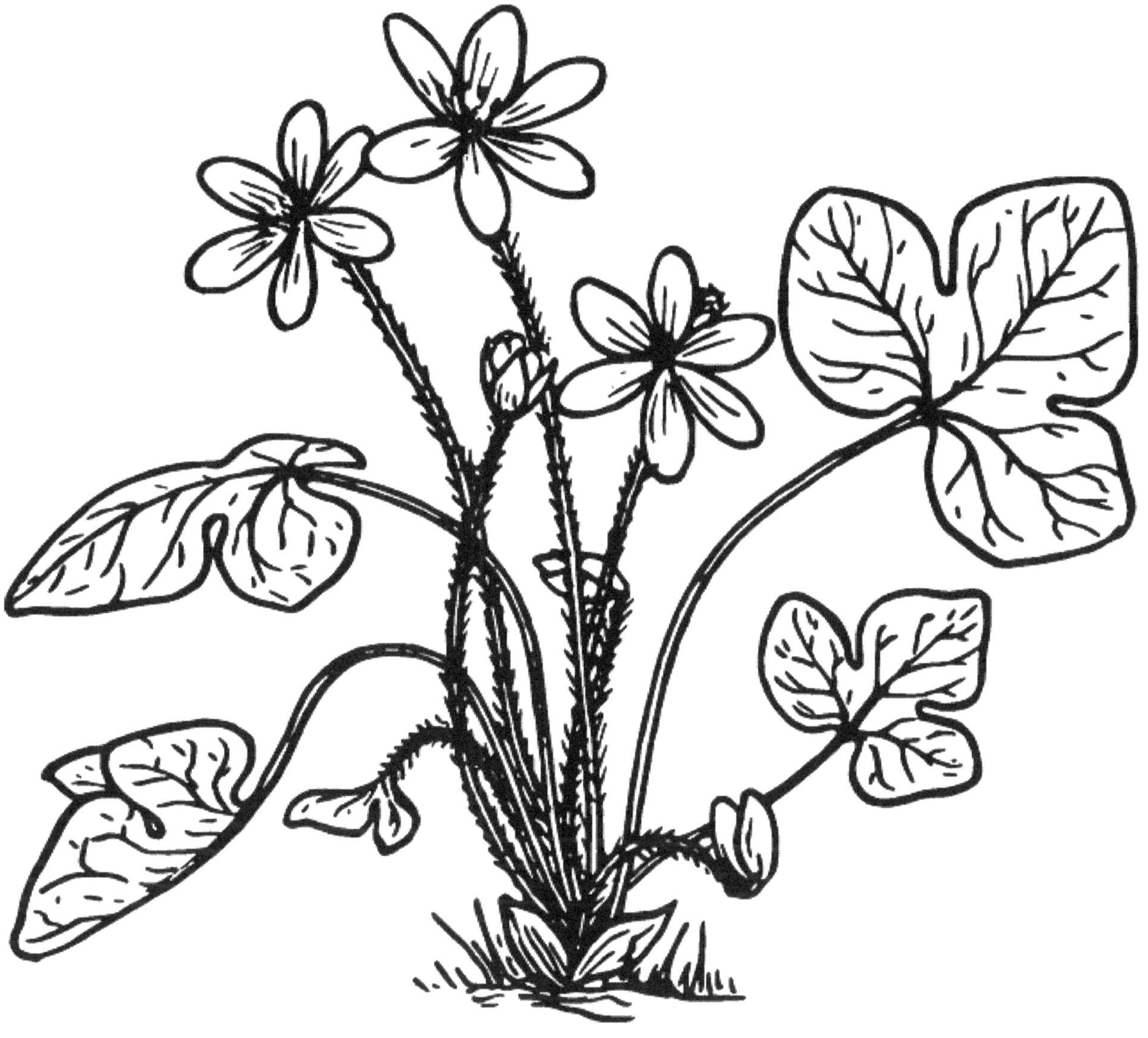

The compounds of a highly respected herbalist incorporate a diverse selection of meticulously chosen herbs that have proven to be highly effective in combating and reversing a multitude of diseases. These compounds have been shown to effectively fight chronic diseases. This individual has talked about the use and benefits of other herbs that are not specifically included in the cell food compounds but are used at their USHA village in Honduras.

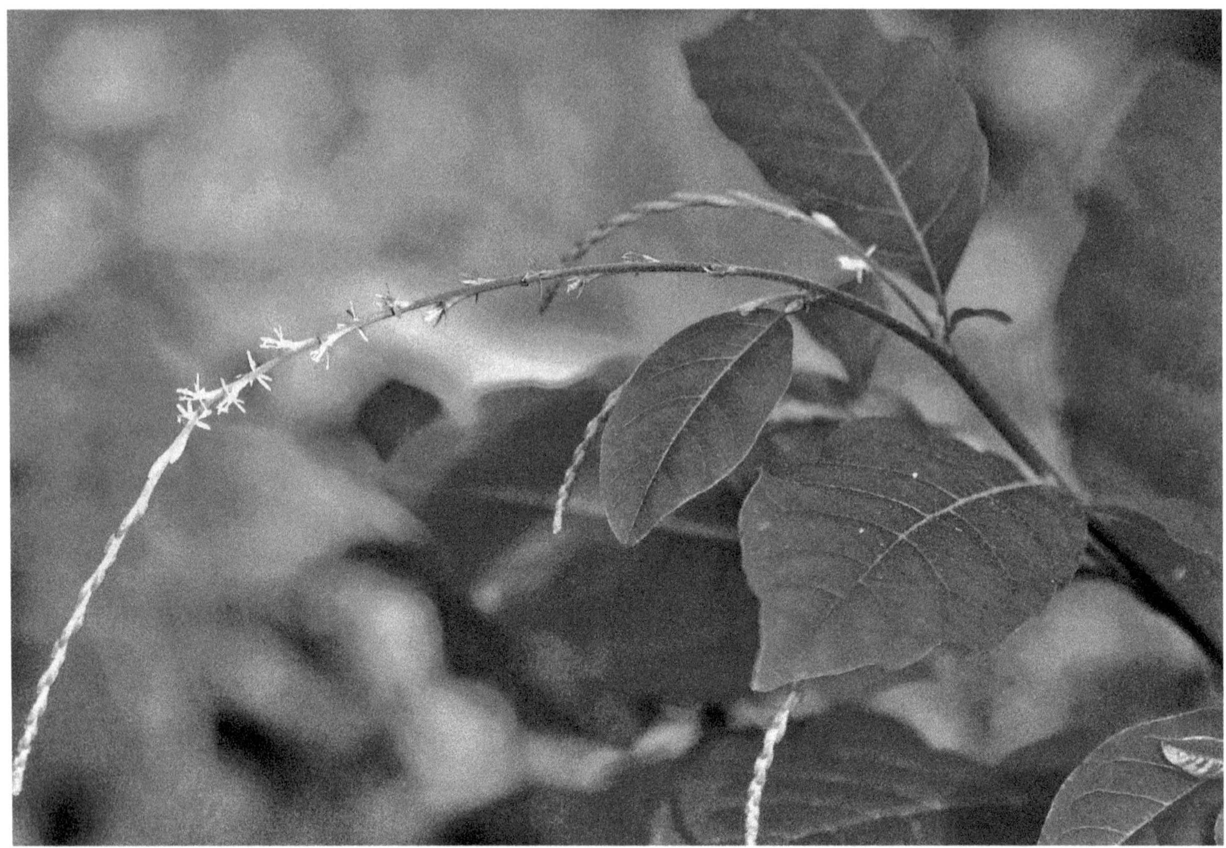

Guinea hen weed, also known as Petiveria alliacea or anamu, is a potent plant that offers a diverse array of health benefits. It has a wide range of beneficial properties, including antimicrobial, anticancer, antitumor, antiviral, antioxidant, diuretic, and anti-HIV effects. Guinea hen weed has a long history in traditional medicine for its potential to address a wide range of health concerns. It has been used for cancer reversal, reducing muscle spasms, lowering fever, promoting nerve relaxation, relieving pain, reducing blood sugar levels, and treating bacterial, fungal, and viral infections.

Origin: The Caribbean, Central and South America General dose: Guinea hen weed is usually consumed as an infusion/tea. 4 oz. of infusion/decoction of leaves and branches, two to three times daily.

Infusion: I tablespoon herb to 8 oz. of boiling water. Steep the herb in the boiling water for I5–20 minutes.

General (capsule) commercial dose: One 500 mg capsule General dosage: One capsule one to two times daily with a meal

Mullein

Mullein, also known as Verbascum, is a versatile plant with a wide range of beneficial properties. It is known for its antiparasitic and antispasmodic effects, as well as its antibacterial, antiviral, anti-inflammatory, antitubercular, and anti-influenza properties. Mullein is commonly used to help clear mucus from the respiratory tract, including the lungs.

Origin: Africa, Asia General commercial dose: One 500 mg capsule

General dosage: Two capsules two or three times daily

CHAPTER 5

HERBAL COMBINATIONS

Combining specific herbs is a common practice to target a particular condition or area of the body. In these situations, the doses are adjusted to be lower than the doses used for the single herbs. While herbs may target similar conditions or body areas, they have distinct approaches. Cells possess receptors that selectively permit the entry of specific nutrients and phytonutrients. Studies have indicated that phytonutrients have the ability to attach to particular receptors found on specific cells. Cells in different regions of an organ may possess distinct receptors for various nutrients and phytonutrients. Take kale, for instance. Its phytonutrients have been linked to a decreased likelihood of developing colon cancer in the middle and right side of the body. On the other hand, apples have been found to be beneficial in reducing the risk of colon cancer in the lower left side of the body.

Unlike pharmaceutical drugs that are artificially created to imitate a single phytonutrient found in a herb or plant, a herb naturally contains a diverse array of phytonutrients that can effectively target various conditions or organs. The nutrients and phytonutrients in a herb function together in a harmonious manner, as opposed to a single nutrient or phytonutrient. The wide range of nutrients and phytonutrients found in a herb, along with their ability to support various functions and organs, is highly beneficial. This is because no organ or metabolic function operates independently from the rest of the body.

Every function is interconnected, and the diverse range of nutrients and phytonutrients found in a single herb contribute to maintaining balance in the body. Certain nutrients and phytonutrients are found in higher concentrations in the herb, while others are found in lower concentrations. This indicates that the herb will have a more potent healing effect in certain areas of the body while its healing effect may be less pronounced in other areas. By combining different herbs, their effectiveness in healing and reversing diseases in specific areas of the body can be enhanced.

NATURAL HERBAL PRODUCTS

An expert in the field of herbalism has been instrumental in distinguishing between top-notch alkaline herbs and the hybrid herbs that are widely available in the market. He has also been incredibly helpful, meticulously putting together herbal packages with precise doses of different herbs to address various ailments. He has simplified the process of identifying the most potent alkaline herbs and determining the optimal dosage.

I have thoroughly explored the characteristics of various herbs found in the packages of this herbalist. Having a comprehensive understanding of the properties and effects of any medication, whether it is traditional or pharmaceutical, is crucial before consuming it. Grasping this concept can also cultivate a favorable outlook on the power of herbs, potentially amplifying their effectiveness through the impact of the mind and suggestion. This phenomenon is often described as the placebo effect, where people achieve positive results because of their strong faith in the treatment.

I have cultivated a strong passion for the field of herbalism and have devoted my time to extensively studying the diverse properties of herbs and their modes of administration. Although herbal medicine is derived from natural plants, the herbs are highly concentrated with phytonutrients and are typically not consumed as food because of their potency. Extensive research has shown the effectiveness of these plant compounds in fighting and reversing different illnesses.

Around half of the pharmaceutical drugs currently in use are synthetic replicas of phytonutrients found in nature. There is a difference between pharmaceutical drugs and individual phytonutrients. Isolated phytonutrients are extracted, synthesized, and concentrated, which boosts their effectiveness but also raises the potential risks linked to their usage. Consuming a large quantity of herbs all at once may cause the body to cleanse too rapidly, which could potentially overwhelm the organs. Nevertheless, the inherent balance and abundance of phytonutrients in herbs typically make their consumption less troublesome.

This expert in herbal medicine has carefully selected combinations that are safe for consumption, promote alkalinity, and can help reverse disease. Here is a complete list of the products available..

CELL PRODUCTS

- Banju
- Bio Ferro
- Bromide Plus
- Estro
- Eva Salve
- Eyewash
- Green Food Plus
- Hair Follicle Fortifier
- Hair food Oil
- Iron Plus

- Testo
- Tooth Powder
- Uterine Wash & Oil
- Viento

PACKAGES

All Inclusive Package: Included Products (20 products): Chelation 1, Chelation 2, Fucus Capsules, Fucus Liquid, L.O.V., Lymphalin, Lupulo, Banju (2), Bio Ferro Tonic (2), Bromide Plus Capsules, Bromide Plus Powder, Bio Ferro Capsules, Green Food, Viento, Iron Plus (2), Endocrine, Testo (for male patients) or Estro (for female patients).

Advanced Package: Products Included (10 products): Chelation 1, Chelation 2, Lymphalin, Fucus Liquid, Lupulo, Bio Ferro Capsules, Bromide Plus Capsules, Viento, Green Food & Iron Plus.

Booster Package: Products Included (7 products): Chelation 2, Lymphalin, Fucus Liquid, Bio Ferro Capsules, Bromide Plus Capsules, Viento & Green Food.

Support Package: Products Included (5 products): Chelation 2, Lymphalin, Bio Ferro Capsules, Bromide Plus Capsules & Viento.

Small Cleansing Package: Chelation2, Bio Ferro and Viento.

It is advisable to consult with a knowledgeable herbalist when using and combining herbs. I have a strong curiosity and enjoy gaining a deep understanding of how things operate.

I have a deep passion for herbalism and the incredible healing properties of plants. As a result, I made the decision to dedicate myself to studying herbs, their unique properties, and the art of combining them. I have shared valuable insights on the effectiveness of specific herbs, their recommended dosage, and how they can be used.

COMBINING HERBS

(This information is intended solely for educational purposes. This information has not been evaluated by the relevant regulatory authority. Please note that the following information is intended for informational purposes only and is not a substitute for professional medical advice. It is crucial to seek guidance from a healthcare professional before making any decisions concerning your health. It's important to remember that the herbs I mentioned have been scientifically proven to have many healing properties. However, their effectiveness is enhanced when used in conjunction with the alkaline plant foods suggested in a well-known herbalist's nutritional guide.

Eating acidic foods like meat, dairy, and processed foods can reduce the effectiveness of these herbs in reversing disease. These herbs have been found to have positive effects on the body's pH levels and can help support the overall well-being of the organs and metabolic functions.

I have created an extensive collection of herb combinations that are carefully designed to target different conditions based on their distinct properties. It is important to drink the recommended one gallon of water daily, as certain herbs can have diuretic properties that may cause dehydration. It's important to make sure you drink enough water to help dilute toxins in your body, which can improve the efficiency of your kidneys and reduce strain on them. It is important to adhere closely to the nutritional guide for maximum health benefits. The foods in the guide offer a wide range of nutrients, phytonutrients, and fiber that help support the body's colon, which is responsible for eliminating solid waste. While there may be some resemblances between these herbal combinations, it's important to note that they are not exact replicas of the curated packages offered by this herbalist.

PARTS

I blend a generous variety of herbs using a conventional method. I carefully store the herbal mixture in a glass jar with a secure lid. I package the herbal blend in 00 standard capsules, each containing around 500 mg of the mixture.

When combining five herbs with a recommended dosage of 500 mg (approximately a quarter teaspoon) each, it is best to mix one cup of each ground or coarsely ground herb together and add the mixture to a jar. This ensures that the herbs are properly blended and ready for use. I use a blender to ensure a thorough mixing of the herbs. I use one cup as the "part" I use. Instead of one cup, I could use a half cup as the portion and combine a half cup of each herb.

I could combine five herbs, with four of them having an individual dose of 500 mg and one of them having a dose of 250 mg. Using one cup as the measurement, I would combine equal amounts of the four herbs, along with a slightly smaller amount of the one herb.

One of the challenges lies in blending herbs with varying dosages. The amount is referred to as the "dose," while the frequency of using the dose is known as the dosage. The recommended dosage for one herb is a 500 mg capsule, which should be taken two capsules two or three times daily. The recommended dose for another herb is a 500 mg capsule, to be taken once or twice daily. The dosage for the second herb would be half of that for the first herb, even though the dose remains the same. This results in using one part of the first herb and one and a half parts of the second herb. Given that both herbs are intended for the same condition, it is not essential to adhere to the complete dosage suggested for each herb. Ensure the herbs are mixed thoroughly and then encapsulate them into 500 mg capsules. Take two capsules two or three times daily.

The herb combinations offered are formulated using 500 mg capsules, which is approximately equal to a quarter teaspoon. The selection of 'part' may differ depending on the desired amount of mixed herb you want to make. You can choose to use either half or one cup as the 'part' or a larger part, depending on the size of your container. I have carefully selected a variety of herbs to offer educational value, offering a glimpse into the skill of blending different herbs together. The herbs used may have similarities to those found in the compounds of a well-known herbalist, although the specific ratios may differ.

Take a moment to explore the details of each herb and discover its unique properties.

THE FOUNDATION

The 'Foundation' is a powerful blend of herbs that efficiently detoxify the liver, kidneys, and blood. These herbs provide a thorough cleansing effect that helps relieve the burden caused by pathogens and toxins on the body's nutrient-delivery system, also known as the blood. Pathogens and toxins can circulate throughout the body, leading to a negative impact on overall health. An imbalanced water-to-electrolyte ratio can have a significant impact on the blood, causing disruptions in electrical activity within cells throughout the body. Improving the liver's ability to remove pathogens and toxins from the blood, and strengthening the kidneys' role in maintaining electrolyte and water balance in the blood. This combination closely resembles the main components found in a well-known herbalist's Bio Ferro.

The Foundation can be used on its own as a versatile cleanser or in combination with other herbal blends. Using multiple combinations together will thoroughly cleanse your body, reaching even the deepest levels.

I part burdock root—Blood purifier, liver cleanser, kidney cleanser I part yellow dock—Blood purifier, liver cleanser, kidney cleanser ½ part sarsaparilla—Binds with toxins I part elderberry—Removes pathogens I part hydrangea root—Breaks up calcification Mix all parts thoroughly in blender.

Make 500 mg capsules or quarter-teaspoon doses.

Dosage: two capsules two or three times daily.

CALCIFICATION REMOVER

Calcification of soft tissue throughout the body hinders the flow of nutrients and phytonutrients to tissue and cells.

Steps

I part hydrangea root—Dissolves kidney stones, cleans lymphatic system ½ part cascara sagrada—Breaks up intestinal waste ½ part red clover —Breaks up waste in lymphatic system, blood purifier Mix all parts thoroughly in blender. Make 500 mg capsules or quarter-teaspoon doses.

Dosage: two capsules two times daily.

PANCREAS AND ENDOCRINE SUPPORT

This blend is known for its ability to support the function of the pancreas and endocrine system, helping to regulate blood sugar levels. It has also shown promise in addressing diabetes. A well-known herbalist includes guaco, huereque, nopal, prodijiosa, and contribo in their 'Endocrine' compound. I decided to leave out contribo from this herbal combination because it can be toxic. It is advisable to seek the guidance of a knowledgeable herbalist when using contribo. I also added sage to the mix.

Steps

½ part guaco—Removes inflammation, mucus, and candida ½ part huereque—Lowers blood-sugar level I part nopal—Reduces type 2 diabetes, high cholesterol, obesity ½ part prodijiosa—Stimulates pancreas secretions, reduces blood sugar level, and induces a vivid dream state I part sage—Lowers glucose level Mix all parts thoroughly in blender. Make 500 mg capsules or quarter-teaspoon doses.

Dosage: three capsules two or three times daily.

GUT AND CELL CLEANSER

The digestive tract is a significant region where numerous diseases can thrive. The digestive tract is home to beneficial bacteria that play a crucial role in supporting the immune system, safeguarding the body from harmful bacteria, fungus, and other organisms. Maintaining a healthy balance of beneficial flora and promoting cell repair in the digestive tract helps to control the growth of harmful fungus like candida.

Candida overgrowth is linked to various gastrointestinal diseases, such as inflammatory bowel diseases (IBD) like Crohn's disease (CD) and ulcerative colitis (UC). Candida is linked to gastric ulcers and lupus, impacting the entire body and leading to conditions such as vaginal yeast infection (candidal vulvovaginitis or vaginal thrush), penis infection (candidal balanitis), and mouth infection (oral candidiasis). These areas can also be affected by herpes outbreaks. These herbs are beneficial for improving the health of the digestive tract, which in turn contributes to overall body balance. This combination can significantly enhance bowel movements, resulting in a frequency of three to six times per day.

An expert in herbal medicine includes cascara sagrada, prodijiosa, and rhubarb root in their chelation 2 product. One of the ingredients in his chelation I formula is blessed thistle. I combine the two elements.

Steps

½ part cascara sagrada—Enhances the overall well-being of the intestines by promoting peristaltic motion to eliminate waste from diverticula; supports the functioning of the stomach, liver, and pancreas Enhances the functioning of the pancreas and liver to support digestion ½ part of rhubarb root is known for its cleansing properties, helping to eliminate heavy metals and harmful bacteria. It is also beneficial for addressing digestive issues and promoting a healthy digestive tract. Includes a component that has been found to have beneficial effects on various bodily functions. These effects include eliminating fungal infections, enhancing digestion, improving blood flow and oxygen supply to the brain, and promoting the health of the heart and lungs. Ensure all parts are mixed thoroughly in the blender. Create capsules with a dosage of 500 mg or quarter-teaspoon measurements.

Recommended dosage: take two or three capsules twice a day.

BRAIN AND NERVE SUPPORT

This combination has a calming effect on nerves and muscles. This mode is specifically tailored to address brain and nerve conditions like attention deficit disorder (ADD) and attention deficit hyperactivity disorder (ADHD). The ingredients in a well-known herbalist's 'Banju' product consist of Santa Maria, blue vervain, burdock root, and elderberry. The 'Foundation' contains ingredients such as burdock root and elderberry, which work effectively with the 'Brain and Nerve Support' to promote a peaceful and optimal state for the brain and nerves.

Steps

I part Santa Maria—Nerve and muscle relaxant, antidepressant I part blue vervain—Heals nerve damage, antianxiety I part tila—Relieves headaches, migraines, inflammation, and depression; relaxes nerves; anticonvulsant I part lavender—Relieves migraines, body pain, and nerve issues; anticonvulsant Mix all parts thoroughly in blender. Make 500 mg capsules or quarter-teaspoon doses.

Dosage: two or three capsules two times daily.

UTERINE SUPPORT (ANTIFIBROID)

This combination provides nourishment to the female endocrine system and helps maintain a healthy balance of estrogen. An imbalance in hormones often leads to the formation of fibroids.

Steps

I part damiana—Balances hormones to shrink fibroids I part hydrangea—Anti-inflammatory, antiseptic, dissolves calcium deposits in soft tissue I part sarsaparilla—Increases sexual desire I part sea moss— Supports connective tissue in vagina ½ part bladderwrack— Antiestrogenic effects lower the risk of estrogen-dependent diseases Mix all parts thoroughly in blender.

Make 500 mg capsules or quarter-teaspoon doses.

Dosage: two to three capsules two to three times daily.

VAGINAL CANAL WASH

Utilize complete portions of herbs. This combination helps to restore the natural balance of flora in the vaginal canal.

Steps

I part arnica flowers—Has antiseptic properties and can help reduce inflammation Red clover is known for its ability to balance estrogen levels and provide relief from menopause symptoms. I part hops—Reduces inflammation Includes sage, which helps balance estrogen levels and provides relief from menopause symptoms. Combine all components. Use a generous tablespoon of mixed herbs.

Infuse one tablespoon of mixed herbs in one cup of boiled water until the water has cooled to room temperature. Filter the herbs, pour the water into a douche bag, and gently apply to the vaginal canal. Recommended for monthly use to maintain optimal performance.

Recommended for use up to three times a week to address vaginal bacterial or fungal conditions.

MALE SUPPORT

An expert in herbal medicine has developed a Testo product that aims to support male health. It contains a blend of natural ingredients including yohimbe, sarsaparilla, sensitiva, and chaparral. I have a special method for blending herbs in my male support formula.

Steps

I part yohimbe (bark, not extract)—Supports libido I part damiana— Supports testosterone balance, relaxes anxiety I part sensitiva—Aphrodisiac, increases sexual desire I part chaparral—Addresses sexually transmitted diseases, cleans cells of penis Mix all parts thoroughly in blender. Make 500 mg capsules or quarter-teaspoon doses.

Dosage: two to three capsules - two times daily

CELL ENERGIZER

This combination is incredibly effective at boosting cellular energy, purifying the body, and rejuvenating overall health. It supports the delivery of oxygen and nutrients to the brain, nervous system, and lymphatic system, while also assisting in reducing cravings for addictive substances. Cell Energizer is similar to a well-known herbal supplement called Iron Plus and Viento. I have removed contribo from the blend in the Viento product. It is crucial to be aware that if contribo is not used correctly, it can potentially harm the kidneys. Therefore, it is advisable to consult with a herbalist for proper guidance when using it. I chose nettle over sea moss.

Steps

I part sapo—Anti-inflammatory, supports kidneys, regulates blood sugar ½ part hombre grande—Antifungal, supports immune system and digestive tract ½ part chaparral—Anti-inflammatory, relieves respiratory issues I part valerian—Relaxes nerves and supports oxygen delivery to the brain I part nettle—General health tonic and blood purifier Mix all parts thoroughly in blender. Make 500 mg capsules or quarter-teaspoon doses.

Dosage: two to three capsules two to three times daily.

NUTRIENT SUPPORT

This supplement is made from natural whole-food sources and is packed with chlorophyll, minerals, vitamins, and phytonutrients.

Steps

I part nettle—Joint support, antioxidant, antimicrobial, nutrient support ½ part tila—Antioxidant, nutrient support I part nopal—Diabetes, nutrient support ½ part bladderwrack—Iodine, nutrient support I part sea moss—Joint and nutrient support Mix all parts thoroughly in blender. Make 500 mg capsules or quarter-teaspoon doses.

Dosage: two or three capsules two to three times daily.

LUPUS BUSTER

Lupus is caused by an overgrowth of candida that leads to a condition known as leaky gut. When food and candida byproducts called mycotoxins enter the bloodstream, they can potentially trigger immune and, over time, autoimmune reactions. An autoimmune disease called lupus can affect various parts of the body, including the central nervous system and joints. These herbal combinations are designed to support the digestive tract, combat candida, and enhance the central nervous system.

- The Foundation
- Gut and Cell Cleanser
- Brain and Nerve Support
- Cell Energizer

COMPLEX DISEASES

Complex diseases such as lupus and cancer are often associated with a disruption of balance in the body. The underlying cause of this breakdown stems from the acidification of the body, leading to the onset of chronic disease.

Chronic disease can present itself in various forms, depending on the specific area of the body that is most affected. Chronic diseases can affect various parts of the body, such as the blood, liver, kidneys, lungs, heart, brain, pancreas, and intestines.

(Please refer to the details about pH in chapter 2.) In contrast to Western pharmaceutical practices and medicine, the African Bio Mineral Balance focuses on healing by restoring balance to the entire body using a variety of nutrients that target different pathways of an illness. On the other hand, Western medicine relies on a single synthetic compound to target a specific issue or symptom. The symptoms of a complex disease are caused by the disruption of multiple processes in the body.

Restoring balance in the body is essential for eliminating all signs of acidification. This is achieved by incorporating alkaline plant foods from a comprehensive nutritional guide and thoroughly cleansing the entire body, including the intracellular level, using a diverse range of herbs.

- The Foundation
- Calcification Remover
- Pancreas and Endocrine Support
- Gut and Cell Cleanser
- Brain and Nerve Support
- Cell Energizer
- Nutrient Support

Female Support

- Uterine Support (Antifibroid)
- Vaginal Canal Wash

Male Support

BLOSSOMS AND OATMEAL FACIAL

This is a simplified version of a product that my sister's soap and body care company produces. Indulge in a luxurious experience for your skin, with the added bonus of being able to customize it with your preferred wetting agent. Plain water is acceptable, but you can elevate the experience by using a hydrosol, yogurt, an egg, milk, or an oil to personalize it.

Ingredients

1 tablespoon rose petals

1 tablespoon yarrow leaves and flowers

1 tablespoon calendula

2 tablespoons oatmeal

Almond meal, cosmetic clay powder, milk powder, or other botanicals (optional)

Directions

Start by placing rose petals in a food processor or, if you prefer, a dedicated coffee grinder for herbs and resins. Break down with a pulse.

Incorporate the remaining ingredients and blend until they reach a relatively consistent texture, similar to the size of grains of sand. Place the mixture into a container that seals tightly.

To use, place approximately a tablespoon of the mixture in a small dish, and incorporate enough of your wetting agent until it reaches a spreadable consistency. After washing your face with your usual cleansing method, gently apply the facial product and massage it onto your skin to provide a mild exfoliation. Keep it on for 5 minutes before rinsing and gently drying

YIELD » 4 OR 5 APPLICATIONS

GARLIC HONEY

This is an exceptional remedy that I prepare during the late summer or early fall, when there is an abundance of local garlic and honey. The honey is absolutely delightful in herbal tea blends, and I can't resist indulging in spoonfuls of garlic cloves.

Ingredients

4 or 5 bulbs garlic

1 pint (470 ml) jar

1 pint (640 g) honey, local preferred

Directions

Take the garlic cloves and carefully remove them from the bulb, making sure to trim off the rough end. After trimming all the cloves, arrange them on a cutting board. Then, using a wide knife held sideways, firmly strike them with the butt of your hand or a fist. This gently mashes them, causing them to be released from their delicate skins. Remove the skins and transfer them into the jar.

Completely cover them with honey. They will reach the pinnacle of the honey, and that's perfectly acceptable. Eventually, they will absorb the honey and sink. Place the covered container in the refrigerator for a minimum of one month.

Rest assured, it will be available whenever you require it.

When you notice the presence of a virus, it's recommended to include a spoonful in a cup of tea. Make sure to repeat this process daily for a few days until the threat has been eliminated.

I always believe that one pint (640 g) at the start of flu season will be sufficient, but I often end up making a second batch in February or March because it never turns out to be enough.

YIELD » 1 PINT (640 G)

PESTO

This easy herb paste is a tasty way to savor the flavors of fresh garlic.

Ingredients

1 cup (60 g) basil leaves

5 or 6 cloves garlic

1 cup (100 g) grated Parmesan cheese

½ cup (75 g) walnuts

¼ cup (60 ml) olive oil

Directions

Place all of the ingredients into a food processor. Blend until creamy or slightly chunky; regardless, it's absolutely delightful when paired with pasta and either shrimp or grilled chicken.

YIELD » 1 CUP (240 G)

HERBS FOR CHILDREN

Children have distinct bodies that differ from adults, with a significantly faster growth rate. Children may metabolize herbs and medications differently than adults, but utilizing herbs for children's health can be highly beneficial and safer than relying on pharmaceuticals. Encouraging the use of homemade natural remedies for kids can often help avoid the use of antibiotics and medications that may have unwanted side effects.

Nevertheless, every situation varies. It is always important to consult with your healthcare provider before introducing herbal interventions for your child.

Create some herbal preparations to help maintain your child's health. Indulge in delicious soups and snacks that are packed with essential nutrients for your well-being.

Utilize herbs to effectively address common ailments in children. For instance, diaper rash, belly aches, teething problems, and minor cuts and bruises can greatly benefit from herbal interventions.

If your child requires traditional medication or therapies, herbs can provide additional support for healing and contribute to overall wellness.

Anise (Pimpinella anisum)

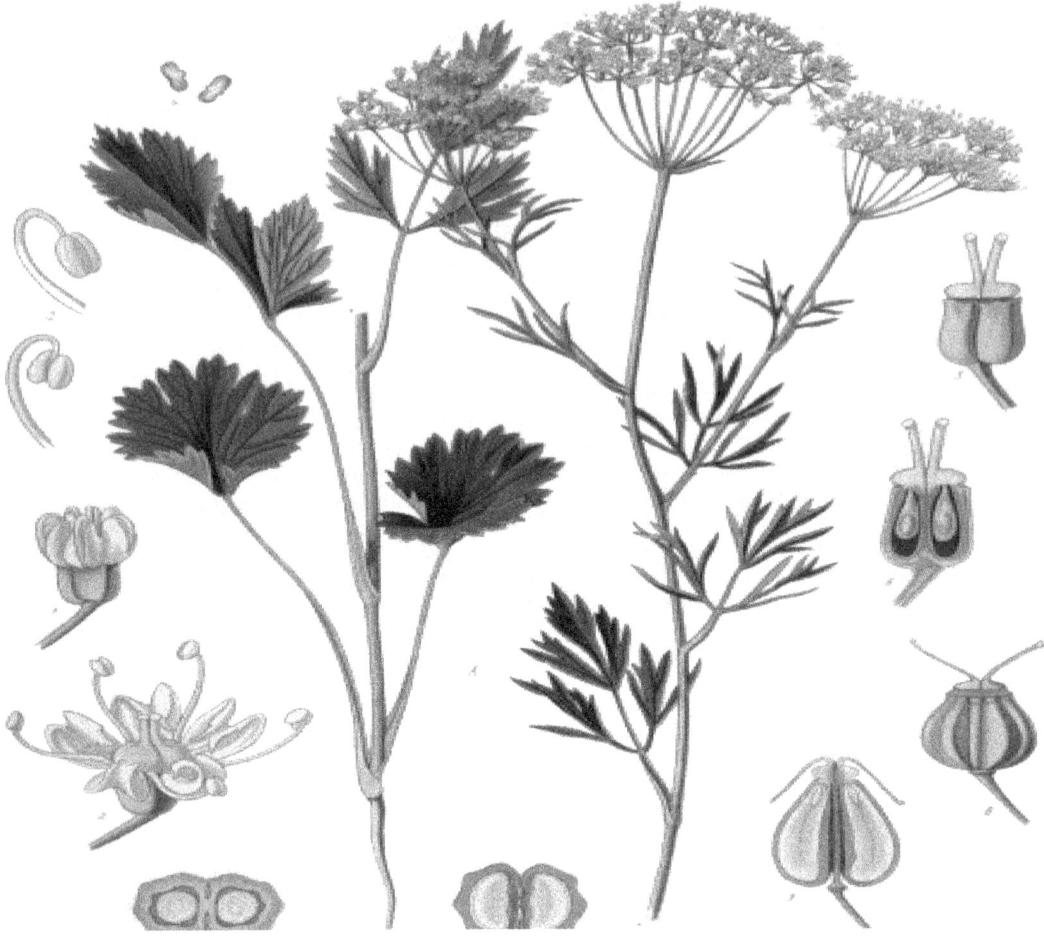

Parts used: primarily the seeds, but the leaves are also useful

Benefits: Anise has a rich historical background as both a medicinal herb and a culinary spice, with a cultivation history spanning over 4,000 years. It is commonly used as a carminative, providing a warming effect and aiding digestion. Additionally, it can provide assistance in addressing mild urinary infections and act as an expectorant for respiratory ailments, aiding in the expulsion of mucus. Most children find the flavor of this product quite enjoyable, with a pleasant licorice-like taste.

Suggested uses: Enjoy this tea for relief from colic and other digestive issues. Due to its delightful taste, anise is frequently combined with less flavorful herbs to enhance their palatability. It creates a delicious syrup.

Astragalus (Astragalus membranaceus)

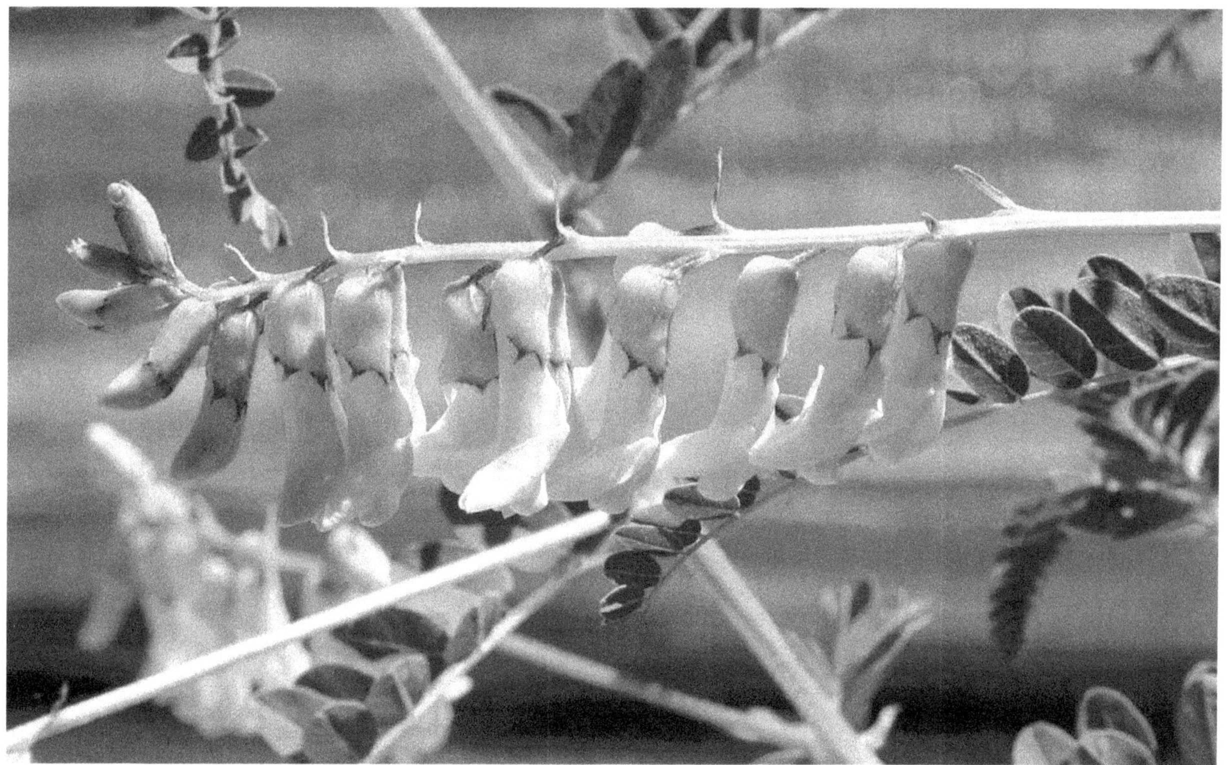

Part used: roots

Benefits: Astragalus is often referred to as the ginseng for the younger generation due to its adaptogenic and toning properties. While echinacea supports the immune system's initial defense, astragalus enhances the deep immune system by aiding in the regeneration of the body's protective shield through the rebuilding of the bone marrow reserve.

Multiple studies have demonstrated the efficacy of this method in supporting young children during chemotherapy and radiation therapy.

Suggested uses: Astragalus is most effective when used in tea to assist patients in recovering from chronic illness and boosting energy levels, while also providing support and strengthening the immune system. The appearance of the root closely resembles the tongue depressors commonly used by doctors, and children may find it enjoyable to chew on, much like a licorice stick. It's possible to include it in soups and broths by adding a root or two (whole or chopped) to the pot and simmering for several hours.

Catnip (Nepeta cataria)

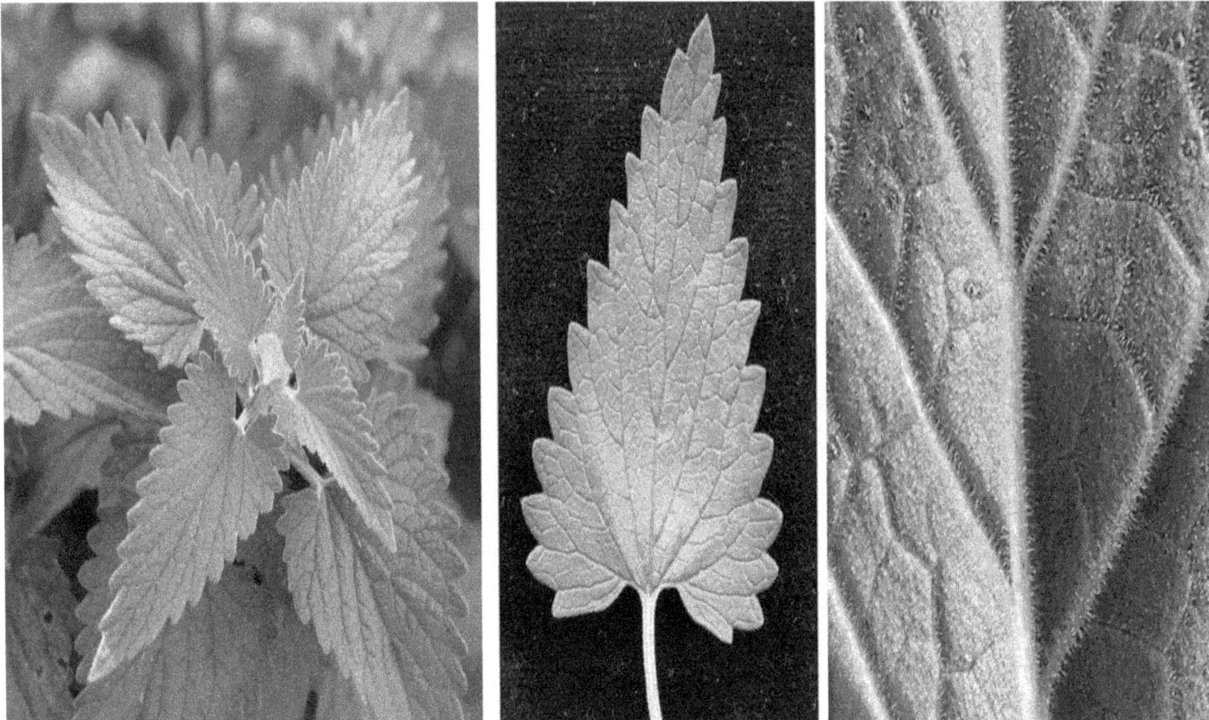

Parts used: leaves and flowers

Benefits: Although catnip may induce euphoria in cats, it is a highly effective herb for humans, known for its calming properties and ability to alleviate various forms of stress. This mode offers exceptional advantages in reducing fever and alleviating the discomfort of teething. Additionally, it serves as a beneficial remedy for digestive issues such as indigestion, diarrhea, and colic. Catnip is a great option for children, as it has calming and relaxing properties. It can also help relieve pain and is gentle on the body.

Suggested uses: Enjoy a soothing cup of tea to help ease teething discomfort at any time of the day. Enhance the flavor of catnip by blending it with herbs like oats and lemon balm, or by incorporating it into fruit juice for a more enjoyable taste. For optimal results, administer a few drops of catnip tincture prior to meals to support healthy digestion. Using a small amount of the tincture before bedtime can help soothe a restless child. This herb is highly effective in reducing childhood fevers. It can be used in both tincture and enema forms for this purpose.

Chamomile (Matricaria recutita, Anthemis nobilis, and related species)

Parts used: primarily the flowers, but the leaves are also useful

Benefits: This small plant possesses incredible healing properties. Its flowering tops contain a significant amount of essential oil, which has potent anti-inflammatory properties. The flowers create a delightfully calming tea that promotes relaxation and aids in digestion. This mode is particularly beneficial for addressing digestive issues that may arise due to stress, such as colic.

Suggested uses: A cup of chamomile tea sweetened with honey can be enjoyed at any time of the day to help soothe a child who is feeling stressed or anxious. An excellent option for achieving a tranquil state and relieving muscle discomfort is a massage oil infused with chamomile essential oil. Adding a small amount of chamomile tincture before meals can help with digestion.

Caution: While chamomile is generally considered safe, it's worth noting that it belongs to the composite family, which can cause allergies in certain individuals. If your child has a high sensitivity or is prone to allergies, it is recommended to conduct a patch test before introducing chamomile to them.

Dill (Anethum graveolens)

Parts used: primarily the seeds, but the leaves are tasty

Benefits: Dill's name is derived from dilla, an ancient Norse term that signifies "to lull." It has gained a notable reputation for its soothing and comforting effects on infants and children. Dill is known for its digestive benefits and is highly regarded for its ability to relieve gas. This herb is widely recognized for its ability to alleviate gastric stress, colic, and nervous digestion in children. Dill is a fantastic source of essential minerals like manganese, magnesium, iron, and even calcium.

Suggested uses: Dill is a popular choice for enhancing the flavors of various dishes. It is also delicious when brewed in tea, either on its own or with other herbs.

Echinacea (Echinacea angustifolia, E. purpurea, and related species)

Parts used: roots, leaves, flowers, and seeds

Benefits: Echinacea enhances the activity of macrophage T-cells, strengthening the body's initial defense against infections. This herb is highly effective in boosting the immune system and combating infections. While this product is powerful and efficient, it is also suitable for children and has been tested to have no adverse effects or lingering residue.

Suggested uses: Echinacea is most effective when used sporadically, rather than on a daily basis. It is recommended to take it when you feel the onset of an infection or when you need to take precautions, such as when everyone at daycare is sick. In such cases, it is advisable to keep your child at home and give her echinacea. When you start feeling under the weather, consider using echinacea in tea or tincture form to strengthen your immune system and potentially prevent the infection. It is most effective when consumed in regular intervals of small amounts. For example, adults would consume a teaspoon of tincture or a cup of tea every 30 to 40 minutes, with the dosage adjusted accordingly for a child. Additionally, it can be beneficial as a tea or tincture for respiratory and bronchial infections in children, and it has the potential to provide relief for sore throats when used in a spray. To alleviate discomfort in your gums and reduce inflammation in your mouth, you can try using the tea or diluted tincture as a refreshing mouthwash. Enhance the flavor with a few drops of peppermint or spearmint essential oil.

Although echinacea is most effective when taken internally, it can also be used externally as a wash or poultice to treat skin infections.

Caution: Similar to chamomile, echinacea belongs to the composite family and can potentially trigger an allergic response in rare cases. If your child is particularly sensitive or prone to allergies, it is advisable to conduct a patch test before introducing echinacea to them.

Important: Due to the high demand for this herb, it has been excessively taken from its natural habitat, leading to its increasing rarity in the wild. It is advisable to avoid echinacea that has been harvested from the wild.

Consider purchasing from reputable companies that offer cultivated echinacea, preferably from organic sources. Even better, cultivate your own.

Elecampane (Inula helenium)

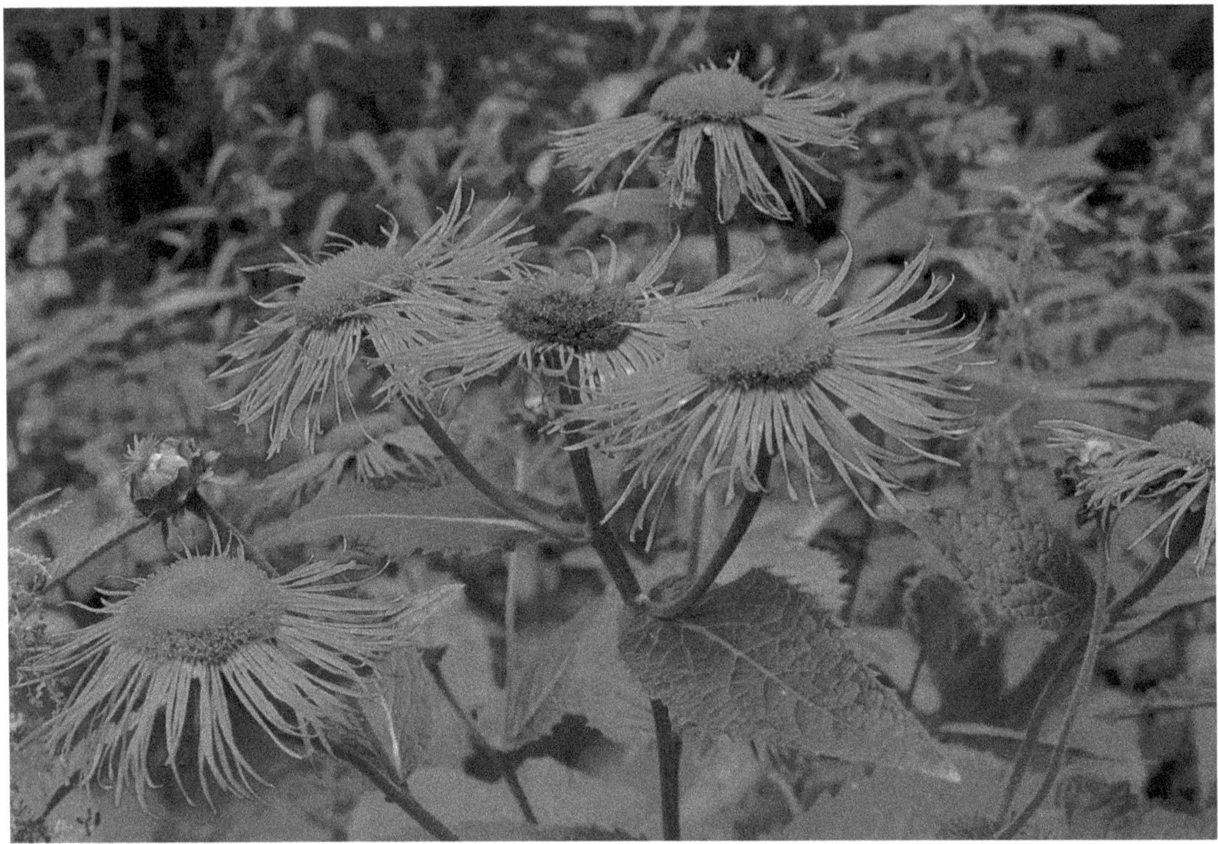

Part used: roots

Benefits: Elecampane is an effective expectorant that helps to clear mucus from the lungs and relieve congestion in the respiratory system. It is a beneficial remedy for coughs, bronchitis, and chronic lung infections. It is particularly potent for coughs when combined with echinacea, licorice, and/or marsh mallow root. If the cough is especially spastic or repetitive, consider incorporating a small amount of valerian, a muscle relaxant, into the mix. If a respiratory or bronchial infection is not responding easily, consider treating it with a mixture of elecampane and pleurisy root. This combination is typically effective for even the most stubborn lung infections.

Suggested uses: Elecampane may not be the most appetizing in terms of taste, so it's important to get creative when serving it to children. As a tea, it can be blended with other delicious herbs like licorice and/or marshmallow root. Enhance the flavor with a touch of cinnamon and add a hint of sweetness using honey or maple syrup. When using the elecampane-pleurisy blend, simply combine the tinctures in equal proportions and enjoy with water, tea, or fruit juice.

Fennel (Foeniculum vulgare)

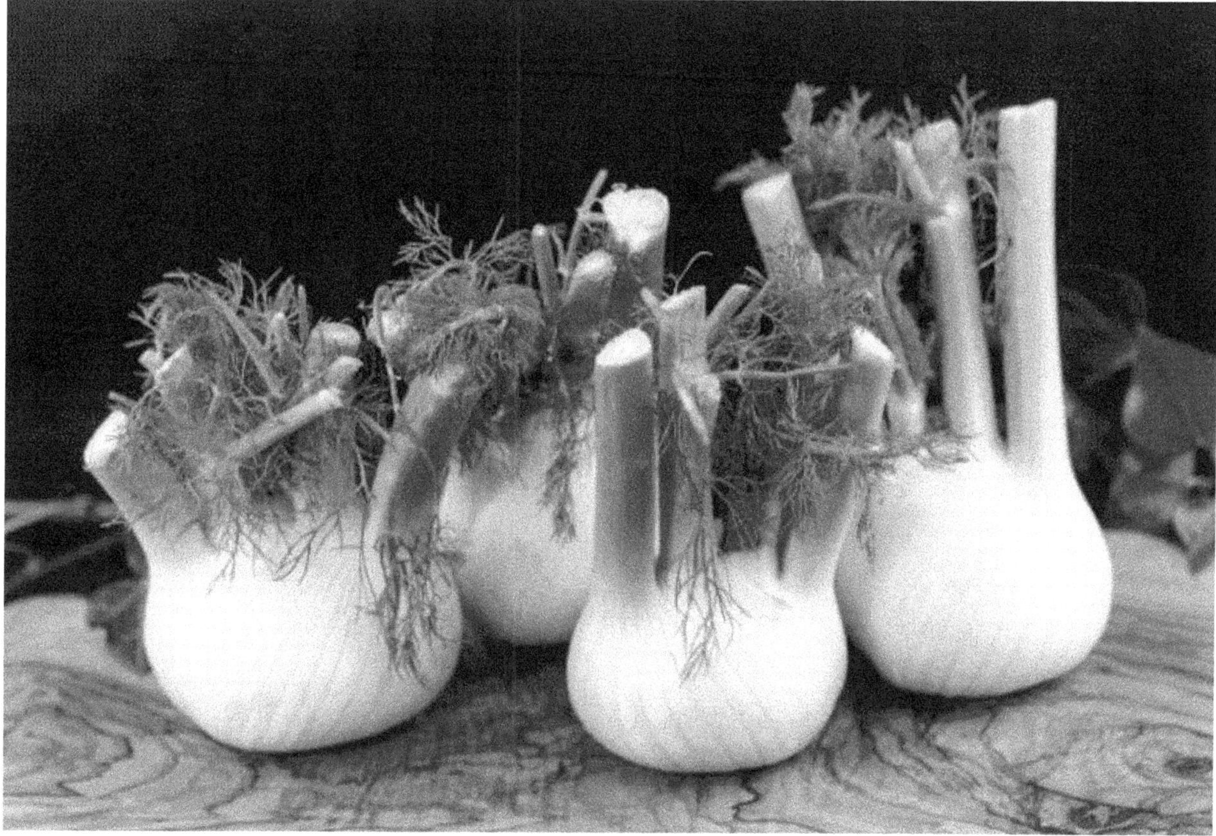

Parts used: primarily the seeds, but the leaves and flowers are also used

Benefits: This plant is famous for its licorice flavor and its reputation as a carminative and digestive aid. It is also well-known for its ability to enhance and nourish the milk supply in breastfeeding mothers. Fennel is a highly effective antacid that can help neutralize excess acid in the stomach and intestines. Additionally, it has the ability to clear uric acid from the joints, which can aid in reducing inflammation and alleviating the pain associated with arthritis. This product is a great digestive aid, helping with digestion, appetite regulation, and relieving flatulence.

Suggested uses: Fennel tea is known for its delicious flavor and its ability to help with colic, digestion, and reducing gas in the body.

For nursing mothers looking to enhance and nourish their milk flow, enjoying two to four cups of tea daily can be beneficial. Additionally, it can be quite helpful in addressing eye inflammation and conjunctivitis. You can try using a warm fennel tea wash that has been carefully strained through a fine-mesh strainer. Due to its delightful licorice-like flavor, fennel is frequently combined with other herbs that may be less flavorful in order to enhance their palatability.

Hawthorn (Crataegus oxyacantha, C. monogyna, and related species)

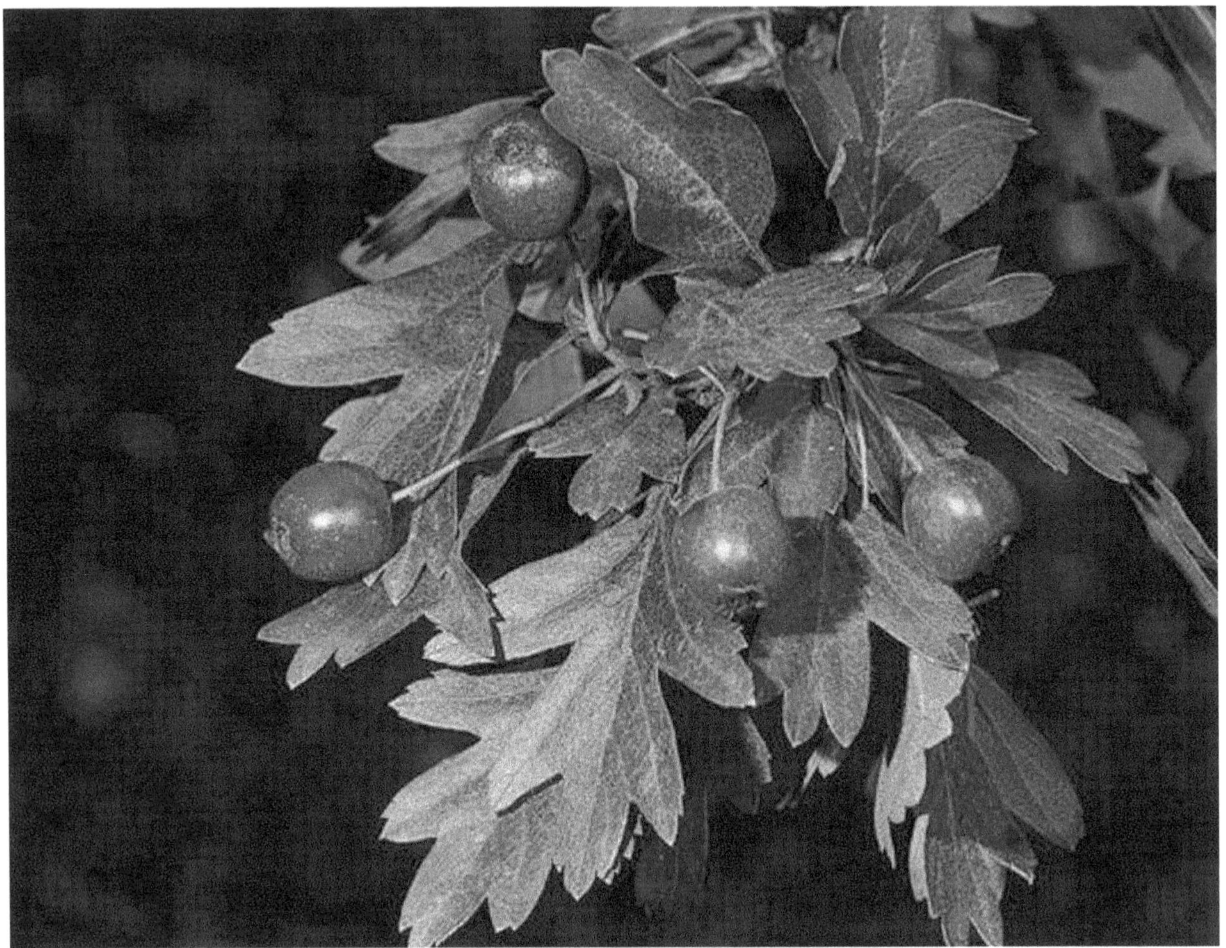

Parts used: fruits, flowers, leaves, and young twigs

Benefits: Hawthorn is known for its antioxidant properties, which can contribute to a strong immune system. It is highly regarded as an exceptional heart tonic, providing strength and nourishment to the heart. Hawthorn is highly effective in promoting heart health and can be used to prevent and treat a range of conditions, including heart disease, edema, angina, and arrhythmia. It can also be beneficial during periods of sorrow and assist us in navigating through the difficult moments of life.

While commonly associated with individuals who have heart conditions or are older, hawthorn is also a beneficial herb for children. It provides essential nutrients for the body, boosts the immune system, promotes healthy vision, and can offer comfort during difficult times.

Suggested uses: Hawthorn can be quite delicious when transformed into a delightful syrup or jam. It can also be enjoyed as a delicious tea when combined with other herbs like hibiscus, oats, and lemon balm. The taste is quite sharp, so it may need to be sweetened. Alternatively, you have the option of using it in tincture form.

Marsh mallow (Althaea officinalis)

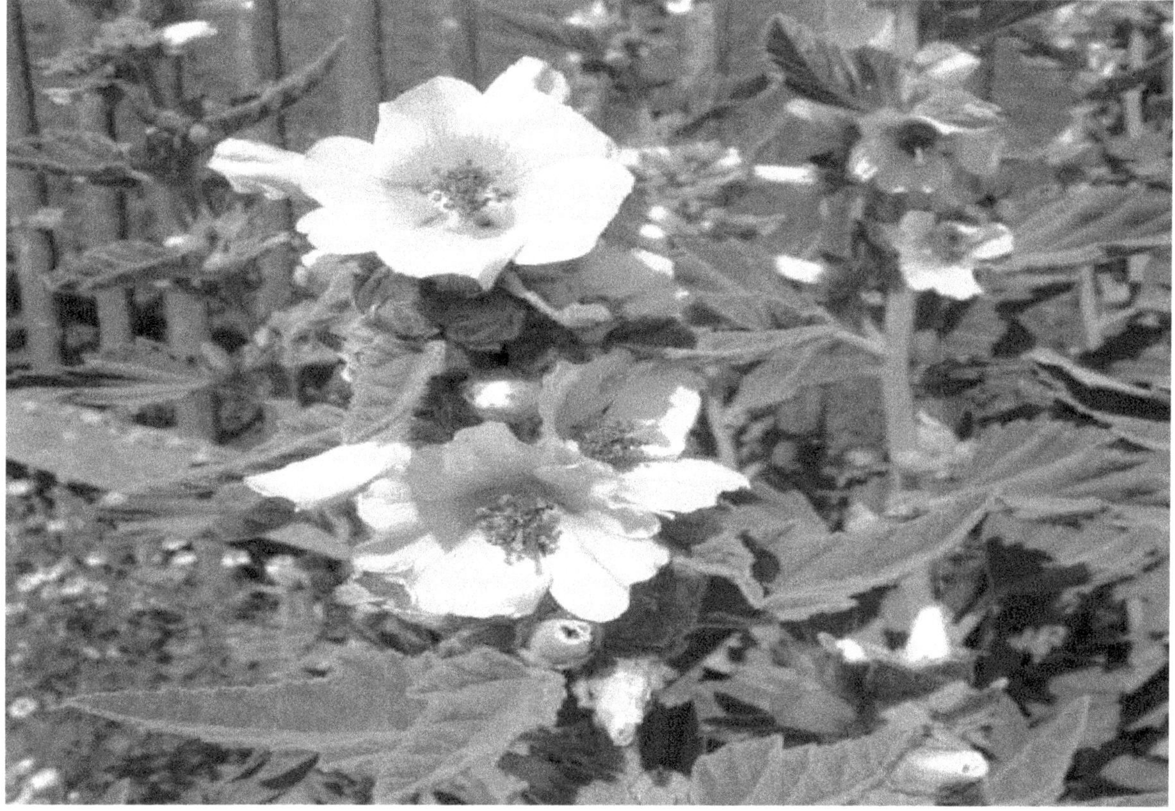

Parts used: primarily the roots, but the leaves and flowers are also useful

Benefits: Marsh mallow is a fantastic alternative to slippery elm when it comes to herbal remedies. It has a soothing and cooling effect, making it a great demulcent. Plus, it's easily accessible and simple to cultivate. Marsh mallow root possesses properties that are both antibacterial and anti-inflammatory. This particular product has a calming effect on inflamed and irritated membranes. It is commonly included in tea blends and tinctures to alleviate symptoms such as sore throat, respiratory infections, and digestive irritation.

Suggested uses: Can be used as a soothing remedy for a sore throat, digestive discomfort, bronchial inflammation, or issues with digestion. Marshmallow is known for its soothing properties on the urinary tract and is often suggested as a natural remedy for urinary tract and bladder infections. Additionally, there are external applications available. You can create a thick paste by mixing it with water to provide relief for burns and irritated skin. Another option is to combine it with oatmeal for a soothing wash or bath to alleviate irritated, itchy dry skin.

Nettle (Urtica dioica)

Parts used: primarily the fresh leaves and young tops, but the roots and seeds are also used

Benefits: Nettle contains a wide range of essential vitamins and minerals. This product is highly beneficial for individuals who require additional iron and calcium. It is commonly recommended for pregnant and nursing mothers to replenish these essential minerals. To enhance its effectiveness, it can be combined with raspberry leaf, which is known for its nutritive properties and its positive impact on female reproductive health. Nettle contains calcium in a highly absorbable biochelated form, making it beneficial for reducing stress and promoting nerve repair. It can be particularly beneficial for the nerves when combined with green milky oats.

Nettle is highly beneficial for supporting tissue and bone repair, often combined with oats and horsetail for this purpose. Due to its rich calcium and mineral content, it aids in promoting strong bone development and can provide relief from growing pains in young children. It is also a highly effective remedy for allergies and hay fever; it has been known to have remarkable results for some individuals. Nettle root is a well-known herb that is highly regarded for its benefits to men's health, particularly in supporting prostate and sexual well-being.

Suggested uses: Nettle has a flavor reminiscent of spinach and is commonly prepared by steaming it and adding a drizzle of olive oil, a squeeze of lemon juice, and a sprinkle of feta cheese. It is often served as a nutritious side dish during meals. It can be a substitute for spinach or other steamed greens in any recipe. However, it needs to be steamed thoroughly to avoid any unpleasant sensations if it's not cooked enough. The tiny hairs found on the underside of the nettle leaf and stems contain formic acid, a substance similar to that found in bee stings. This can cause the skin to swell and result in an uncomfortable, irritating rash. When picking nettles, it's important to wear gloves and be cautious not to come into contact with it. Additionally, it's crucial to educate your children about the importance of respecting this plant. If someone happens to get "stung," they can apply a plantain leaf poultice to draw out the toxins.

Freeze-dried form appears to be the most effective way to use nettle for allergies, whether as a tincture or tea. For optimal results, consider combining freeze-dried nettle capsules with nettle tea and/or tincture. This combination can enhance the overall effectiveness.